Work-Based Learning

Level 3

**AWARD
CERTIFICATE
& DIPLOMA**

DEMENTIA

Yvonne Nolan

ALWAYS LEARNING

PEARSON

Published by Pearson Education Limited, Edinburgh Gate, Harlow, Essex, CM20 2JE.

www.pearsonschoolsandfecolleges.co.uk

Heinemann is a registered trademark of Pearson Education Limited

Text chapter 1 © Nicki Pritchatt
Text chapters 2-5 © Yvonne Nolan
Typeset by Tek-Art, Crawley Down, West Sussex
Original illustrations © Pearson Education 2012
Illustrated by Tek-Art, Crawley Down, West Sussex
Cover design by Pearson Education 2012
Picture research by Emma Whyte
Cover photo/illustration © Plainpicture Ltd: Johner

The right of Yvonne Nolan and Nicki Pritchatt to be identified as authors of this work have been asserted by them in accordance with the Copyright, Designs and Patents Act 1988.

First published 2012

16 15 14 13 12
10 9 8 7 6 5 4 3 2 1

British Library Cataloguing in Publication Data

A catalogue record for this book is available from the British Library

ISBN 978 0 435 07787 7

Printed in Spain by Grafos S.A.

Every effort has been made to contact copyright holders of material reproduced in this book. Any omissions will be rectified in subsequent printings if notice is given to the publishers.

Websites
Pearson Education Limited is not responsible for the content of any external Internet sites. It is essential for tutors to preview each website before using it in class so as to ensure that the URL is still accurate, relevant and appropriate. We suggest that tutors bookmark useful websites and consider enabling students to access them through the school/college intranet.

Contents

Acknowledgements

The publisher would like to thank the following for their kind permission to reproduce their photographs:

(Key: b-bottom; c-centre; l-left; r-right; t-top)

Alamy Images: Adrian Sherratt 73, amana images inc 70, Blend Images 29b, Colin Underhill 86, Corbis Flirt 76, Dan White 25, Fancy 38, Golden Pixels LLC 29t, gulfimages 107, Mark Wiener 27, NewStock 106, Paula Solloway 55, Robert Nicholas 54; **Corbis:** Michael Haegele 39, Ocean 103; **Getty Images:** Digital Vision 12, Terry Vine / Blend 104; **Pearson Education Ltd:** Lord and Leverett 50, 51, Richard Smith 102b; **Plainpicture Ltd:** Fancy Images 65t, Image Source 6, mia takahara 19, Senior Images 53, Susan Kirch 17; **Shutterstock.com:** Alexander Raths 10, auremar 102t, AXL 41, corepics 58, Dmitry Kulagin 85, IDAL 23, lightpoet 75, Monkey Business Images 14, 65b, Paul Aniszewski 63, Yuri Arcurs 11, 33, 71; **SuperStock:** Stock Connection 4, Yuri Arcurs / SuperFusion 16; **www.TalkingMats.com:** 49

Cover images: *Front:* **Plainpicture Ltd:** Johner

All other images © Pearson Education

We are grateful to the following for permission to reproduce copyright material:

Text on page 48 of suggestions for supporting communication with people who have dementia from Bryden, C. (2012). *Who will I be when I die?* Jessica Kingsley Publishers, London and Philadelphia. Reprinted with permission of Jessica Kingsley Publishers; List of personal enhancers and detractors on pages 50–51, from *Brooker, C. (2006) Person-centred Dementia Care: Making Services Better. Jessica Kingsley Publishers, London and Philadelphia.* Reprinted with permission of Jessica Kingsley Publishers.

In some instances we have been unable to trace the owners of copyright material, and we would appreciate any information that would enable us to do so.

How to use this book

Welcome to the Level 3 book to accompany the Dementia units for health and social care. The content of this book is intended to meet your needs if you are studying for the Award in Awareness of Dementia, the Certificate in Dementia Care or the Dementia pathway of the Diploma in Health and Social Care.

This book covers five topics:

1   understanding the process and experience of dementia

2   administration of medication

3   communication

4   equality, diversity and inclusion

5   enabling rights and choices.

Two of these topics cover both a knowledge unit and a competence unit. This is because much of the content of the units is usually identical. In the margins of these chapters, you will see that it clearly signposts which criteria are covered in each section. To make it easy to track, the knowledge unit references are in **red** and the competence unit references are in **blue**.

For example:
AC **310:1.2** and **313:1.1**

This section covers assessment criteria 1.2 from the knowledge unit and 1.1 from the competence unit.

You may find that you do not need to look at these references, but you can be sure that all the assessment criteria for the topics are covered in this book.

Special features

Look out for the following special features as you work through the book.

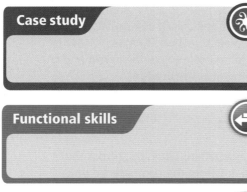

Case study

Real-life scenarios that explore key issues and broaden your understanding

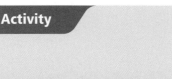

Functional skills

This indicates where you can demonstrate your English, mathematics or ICT skills

Activity

A pencil and paper icon marks opportunities for you to consolidate and/or extend learning, allowing you to apply the theoretical knowledge that you have learned in health and social care situations

Doing it well

Information around the skills needed to perform practical aspects of the job. These are often in the form of checklists that you can tick off point by point to confirm that you are doing things correctly

Reflect

Reflect features have thought bubbles, to remind you that they are opportunities for you to reflect on your practice

Key term

Look out for the keyhole symbol that highlights these key terms – clear definitions of words and phrases you need to know

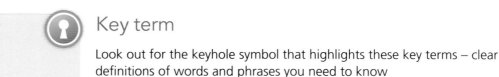

Getting ready for assessment

Information to help you prepare for assessment, linked to the learning outcomes for the unit

Further reading and research

Useful for continuing professional development, including references to websites, books and agencies

Understand the process and experience of dementia

This unit provides you with the knowledge you need on the neurology of dementia, including the causes of dementia and the difficulties and needs of the person with dementia. This knowledge will help to support your understanding of how people may experience dementia.

With the development of improved health care and healthier lifestyles, people are living longer. With an increase in an ageing population come age-related conditions such as dementia. Age is one of the major risk factors of developing dementia.

In this unit you will learn about:

■ the neurology of dementia
■ the impact of recognition and diagnosis of dementia
■ how dementia care must be underpinned by a person-centred approach.

1: The neurology of dementia

1.1 Causes of dementia

The word 'dementia' is a term that describes a serious deterioration in mental functions, such as memory, language, orientation and judgement. There are over 100 different causes of dementia. In this chapter we will cover the main causes of dementia.

The brain is a complex organ and is divided up into different areas that control different functions within the body. The brain contains around 100 billion cells. In dementia some of these cells stop working properly. The part of the brain that this occurs in will affect how that person thinks, remembers and communicates.

Dementia is a major health condition which affects over 820,000 people in the UK. Worldwide, more than 35 million people are estimated to have dementia, with 4.6 million new cases being diagnosed every year. It is a global problem that has a significant socioeconomic impact. In this country alone, the cost of dementia care is currently around £8 billion a year in direct care costs, and it is believed the cost could triple in the next 20 years (source: Health Foundation, 2011).

Types of dementia

Alzheimer's disease

Many people ask if dementia and Alzheimer's disease are the same thing. The short answer is no. Alzheimer's disease is the most common cause of dementia. It is responsible for approximately two-thirds of dementia in older people. Alzheimer's is caused by nerve cells dying in certain areas of the brain. In addition to this, the connections between affected nerve cells deteriorate. As the disease progresses, it spreads and affects cells in other parts of the brain.

Vascular dementia

Vascular dementia is a form of dementia caused by damage to the brain due to deprivation of oxygenated blood. It is the second most common form of dementia. Oxygenated blood is carried around your body and brain through arteries. Deoxygenated blood is carried through your body in veins. These arteries and veins make up your vascular system. When an

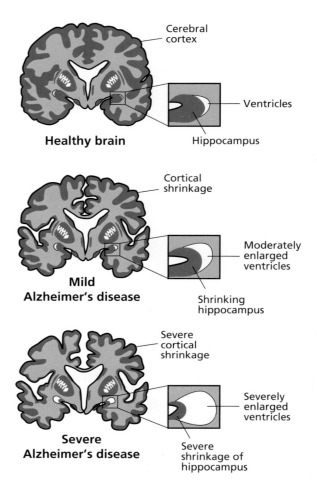

Figure 1.1: Brain affected by dementia and unaffected brain

organ in your body is deprived of blood, that organ (or part of it) will die. This is what happens to the brain in vascular dementia.

Individuals often experience stroke-like symptoms, so physical problems alongside the symptoms of dementia are common. Deterioration normally takes place in stages, and depression is common in this type of dementia.

The conditions which can cause vascular dementia are preventable and include high blood pressure, heart problems, diabetes and high cholesterol. When supporting people into leading a healthy lifestyle, it is important to bear this condition in mind, in the hopes of preventing the onset of vascular dementia. Particular communities that are at higher risk of high blood pressure such as the Afro-Caribbean communities are more at risk of this type of dementia. Individuals can have both vascular dementia and Alzheimer's disease at the same time; mixed presentations are common.

Dementia with Lewy Bodies (DLB)

Lewy Bodies are tiny spherical protein deposits which are found inside the nerve cells of the brain. These deposits alter the way the brain functions and can be found in people with both dementia and Parkinson's disease. Approximately four per cent of the older population who have dementia are affected by DLB, and it is the third most common form of dementia. This kind of dementia is characterised by motor skills difficulties, for example, difficulty with walking, spatial orientation and hallucinations, although hallucinations can also be experienced in other types of dementia. Individuals with DLB are often over the age of 65 and can present with moments where they are very lucid (or less confused).

Rarer forms of dementia

Fronto-temporal dementia

Fronto-temporal dementia is a rare form of dementia. It tends to affect younger people and is more common among men. The condition is caused by damage to the frontal lobe and/or the temporal parts of the brain. These areas are responsible for the person's behaviour, emotional responses and language skills. Types of fronto-temporal dementia include Pick's disease, frontal lobe degeneration and dementia associated with motor neurone disease.

Creutzfeldt-Jakob disease (CJD)

CJD is a form of dementia caused by prion disease. Prions are proteins which are found in mammals. When these proteins cluster together in the brain, they cause brain cells to die. When these cells die they leave holes in the brain called spongiosis. When examining the brain under a microscope, the cells appear sponge-like. This damage to the brain causes neurological difficulties and dementia.

There are four forms of CJD:

1 sporadic
2 familial
3 iatrogenic
4 variant.

Although each of these conditions is very rare, their prognosis is extremely poor. The affected person's life expectancy is radically reduced, with death occurring usually within 6 to 24 months from early diagnosis. The disease can take many years from the time it infects a person to it causing recognisable symptoms.

The cause of sporadic CJD is unknown and its onset is very fast. It affects people over the age of 50 and can cause death within a matter of months.

Familial CJD is an inherited form of the disease. Its symptoms usually affect the person at an early age, from 20 to 60 years. Death occurs between two and ten years of symptoms beginning.

Iatrogenic CJD occurs as a result of contaminated blood or tissue entering the healthy person's body. This can take place with corneal transplants, grafts or the use of growth hormones. To prevent the risk of contamination, transplants are no longer taken from people known to have the disease and growth hormones are now developed artificially. Because prions cannot be destroyed using normal sterilisation procedures, any surgical instruments used on people with CJD are not used on other patients.

The last form of CJD is known as variant CJD. This form affects people at a younger age, with the average age of death being 29 years. The average time the person is affected by this disease is 14 months. Variant CJD is caused by bovine spongiform encephalopathy (BSE) – a form of prion disease which affects cattle. The person contracts this disease by eating infected beef products. To greatly reduce the risk of infected beef products reaching the market, manufacturers now remove the animal's brain and spinal cord from general sale.

> **Functional skills**
>
> **Maths: Recording data**
>
> This information can be used to record data in a chart and to show the use of working out averages for statistical purposes.

Biswanger's disease

This is a form of vascular dementia in which damage occurs to the blood vessels in the deep white matter of the brain. It affects people over the age of 60 and is often a result of long-term hypertension or high blood pressure.

Dementia and learning disabilities

Some people with learning disabilities are at risk of developing dementia in adult life. There is a higher risk of dementia in the general learning disability population, and it is more prevalent in individuals with a diagnosis of Down's syndrome. The risk of Alzheimer's increases as the person gets older. It is estimated that over half of the people with Down's syndrome will develop Alzheimer's disease when they are in their 60s.

1.2 Memory impairment and dementia

With regard to humans, the term 'memory' refers to information stored in the brain, and to the retention (keeping) and recalling of that information. A person's brain is extremely complex and can store, retain and recall many, many pieces of information for many, many years. The ease with which a person can remember information will vary depending on the subject, the person and their state of mind.

There are three main categories of memory: sensory memory, short-term memory and long-term memory.

Short-term memory

Short-term memory temporarily records information but has a very limited span of less than a minute. It can only store about seven items. It may register a face that we see in the street or a telephone number that we overhear someone giving out, but this information will quickly disappear forever unless we make a conscious effort to retain it.

Short-term memory is significant, as we need to hold on to information long enough to work out what to do with it – for example, remembering a conversation so that we know how to respond, or making a calculation work. We commit things from short-term to long-term memory by repetition, i.e. by recalling them frequently. Our interest and motivation also play a part. For example, we are more likely to transfer things to long-term memory that link to other ideas we already have or things that are of interest to us.

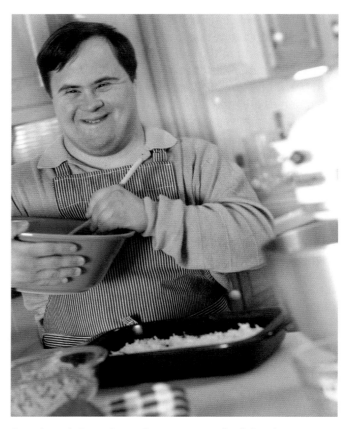

People with Down's syndrome are at risk of developing Alzheimer's disease.

Short-term memory is frequently affected in people who have dementia. If someone starts to experience memory problems and this is accompanied by problems with other thinking or planning skills, it is possible that they are developing a form of dementia. Memory loss alone does not constitute dementia.

Long-term memory

Long-term memory stores all the information and events that we can recall, including the physical skills that we have learned. Its storage capacity can last a very long time, even a lifetime. As we grow older long-term memory can become affected.

The three main categories of long-term memory are semantic, episodic and procedural memory. Each of these types of long-term memory has a different function. People who have damage to these types of memory will present in different ways.

Semantic memory enables us to recall facts such as the capital of a city or the name of the place where we live. If this part of memory is impaired, the individual with dementia will find it difficult to recall words or names of objects.

Episodic memory enables us to recall events and experiences in our lives. Often significant events in life are well rehearsed in our minds, making them easier to recall (times, places, associated emotions and other contextual knowledge). Often when we recall episodic events there is an emotional response alongside the memory, and so this type of memory is more than just the facts surrounding the event. Emotions and memories are interlinked, and consideration needs to be given to this when carrying out reminiscence-type training that aims to recall episodic memories.

Procedural memory enables us to carry out motor tasks such as riding a bike, signing our name or driving a car. This type of memory is often retained for longer. This type of memory is implicit – this means that it is unconscious, so often there is no conscious thought about carrying out these actions. Patients with profound amnesia often retain procedural memory.

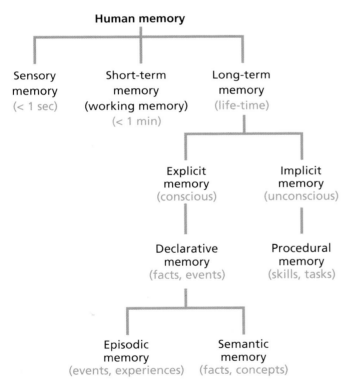

Figure 1.2: Organisation of the human memory

Types of memory loss

As you get older, you can have a natural amount of memory loss. If this is significant the clinical name for it is mild cognitive impairment. This is different to dementia as damage is only in the area of memory.

Functional skills

English: Writing; Reading

In this book there are a number of case studies. These studies have all been laid out using a suitable format and attention has been paid to ensure that spelling, punctuation and grammar are accurate. You will need to use these skills when writing case studies in your place of work. You will need to read and understand both straightforward and complex texts, and use the information in an appropriate way.

Short-term memory loss

Short-term memory can differ from one person to another. Research into differences in short-term memory has been carried out on this by asking people to remember numbers. A list of numbers is read out at approximately one number per second. The person is then asked to recall these numbers. The results of this research show that on average a person can remember seven consecutive numbers.

A person with dementia may have difficulties remembering things that happened only a short while ago. However, the same person may be able to remember things that happened many years ago. Other memory difficulties could include:

- a difficulty in recognising people or remembering their names
- the inability to find the right words for things or objects
- repeating conversations that they have already had
- asking the same question again in a short space of time
- forgetting appointments or recent events
- misplacing items, forgetting where they have put things or where they are usually kept
- the inability to recall what they have had to eat or even forgetting they have eaten
- the loss of skills such as self-care, washing, dressing, putting clothes on in the right order, shopping and cooking
- the inability to judge time – for example, thinking it is time to get up when it is the middle of the night
- forgetting where they live
- becoming unaware of their surroundings

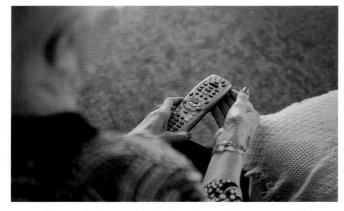

How do you think it might feel to be unable to remember the word for this object?

- forgetting to take medication, possibly thinking they have already taken it
- forgetting their disabilities – for example, getting up to walk even though they are not able, which results in them falling
- an inability to have empathy, which could make the person appear selfish.

Initially people experiencing these memory losses may feel frustrated or angry with themselves. They are angry because they know that they have forgotten, and frustrated because they are unable to remember as they used to.

Activity 1

Memory impairments

Think about the people you support. What types of memory difficulties do they experience and how do you know about this?

Functional skills

English: Speaking and listening

Have a discussion with colleagues about the types of memory difficulties that people you are working with have. Ensure you take an active part in the discussion and that you show effective listening skills.

It is important to keep in mind that no two people's memories will be affected by dementia in the same way. The inappropriateness of their behaviours is caused by a physical change to the brain and therefore the person has no control over it.

1.3 How individuals process information with reference to the abilities and limitations of individuals with dementia

The workings of the brain are very complex. As stated previously, the human brain is made up of around 100 billion cells. In the main these cells are called neurons. It may be easier to think of these neurons as switches which are either switched on or switched off. If the neuron is switched off it is resting; when it is switched on it fires electrical impulses along its body, which is called the axon. At the end of the axon there is a small part that releases a chemical. The chemical travels over a gap called the synapse and turns on another neuron. These chemicals are called neurotransmitters. There are 60 identified chemicals involved in the brain's activity.

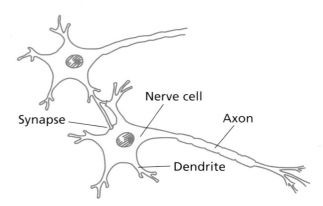

Figure 1.3: The amount of electricity the human brain produces when each of its neurons is firing is equivalent to a 60-watt light bulb.

Types of neurotransmitters

The following are some important neurotransmitters relating to the process of memory and associated functions.

Reading about these chemicals and what they do will help you understand how the person with dementia, who has damage to these neurons, has difficulty with their memory. Because the neurons are damaged or destroyed, they are not able to produce or transmit important chemicals which are required for the person to function fully.

Dopamine

The chemical dopamine is critical for controlling your body's movements. If you do not have enough dopamine, you will not be able to move or control your movements very well. Dopamine also controls the flow of information from other areas of the brain, especially memory, attention and problem-solving tasks.

Serotonin

The chemical serotonin is the neurotransmitter enhanced by many antidepressants, such as Prozac, and has become known as the 'feel-good' neurotransmitter. It has a profound effect on mood, anxiety and aggression.

Acetylcholine (ACh)

ACh controls activity in the areas of the brain that are connected with attention, learning and memory. People with Alzheimer's disease tend to have low levels of ACh in their brain.

Glutamate

Glutamate is vital for making the links between neurons that are the centre of learning and long-term memory.

Left and right sides of the brain

The collection of 100 billion cells or neurons in the brain is divided into two halves, which are called the hemispheres of the brain. The right side of the brain is responsible for putting information together – for example, information received from your eyes. If you see a lady, the information goes from your eyes to the right side of your brain, firing neurons which put the information together, so you are able to say, 'I can see a lady.' The left side of the brain analyses information which is collected by the right side of the brain. It enables you to expand on what you see so you are able to say, 'I know who that lady is. It's my sister Michelle.'

People with dementia who have damage to the neurons on the right side of the brain will have difficulty putting information together. They will be able to 'see' things, items or people, but will not be able to make the connection as to what those things, items or people are.

People with dementia who have damage to the neurons on the left side of the brain tend to be affected by depression. They will have more organisational problems and will have problems using language.

Different parts of the brain are responsible for different cognitive skills. When receiving information into the brain the brain uses the relevant sensory parts of the brain to identify and associate this to what it already knows, and then it works out how the person should respond. Where there is damage, information coming into the brain will be misperceived and therefore the response or action from the person with dementia may not be appropriate. This can sometimes lead to breakdown in communication and may put the person at risk in certain situations.

1.4 How other factors can cause changes in an individual's condition that may not be attributable to dementia

There are a number of other conditions which can be confused with dementia. It is important that support workers identify these, as many of them can be treated to improve the quality of life for the person with dementia.

Depression

Depression is common among people with dementia, so it is possible for a person to have both dementia and depression. Depression can often be treated using either medical or non-medical interventions. Depression can present in the following ways which could be confused with dementia:

- lack of motivation
- excessive sadness
- not sleeping well at night
- lack of appetite
- memory problems
- difficulty concentrating
- slow thought processes and speech.

Delirium

Some of the things that cause **delirium** are:

- systemic infections (especially urinary tract and chest infections)
- vitamin B deficiencies
- liver or kidney failure
- hydrocephalus (increased pressure in the brain that squashes neural tissue)
- dehydration
- intoxication through drugs or alcohol.

> **Key term**
>
> **Delirium** – severe confusion, involving rapid changes between different mental states and disorganised thinking.

People suffering from delirium can present with dementia-like symptoms, including:

- poor concentration
- fluctuating consciousness
- language disturbance
- disorientation
- seeing things differently (perceptual difficulties).

Delirium is common in older people because of underlying physical problems. However, these symptoms can often be treated simply through the application of medical treatments.

Mild cognitive impairment (MCI)

Mild cognitive impairment (MCI) is a relatively new term to describe those who show some difficulties with their memory but do not have dementia. Studies have shown that 50 per cent of people with MCI go on to develop dementia later in life.

Brain injury

Injuries to the brain can be caused by external trauma such as a blow to the head, or internal factors such as a stroke or aneurysm. The level of brain injury can be anything from mild to severe. It can result in short-term, long-term or permanent difficulties.

Brain tumour

A tumour of the brain can be benign (slow-growing, non-cancerous) or malignant (invasive, often growing rapidly and cancerous). It can affect memory and other functions such as speech, communication and concentration. A brain tumour can also cause personality changes and confusion.

Medication

Some prescription medications such as anticholinergic and antipsychotic medications can have side effects which can affect somebody's memory.

Hydrocephalus

Hydrocephalus is usually associated with spina bifida and is caused by a build-up of cerebro-spinal fluid (CSF) in the brain. This condition can also be caused by infections such as meningitis, premature birth, head injury or stroke. Hydrocephalus can lead to problems with concentration, short-term memory, organisation and coordination.

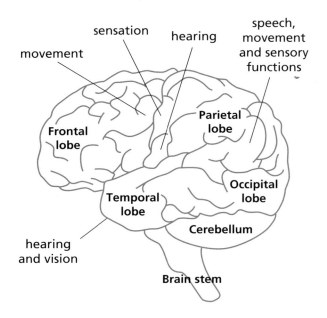

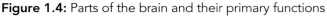

Figure 1.4: Parts of the brain and their primary functions

Lack of sleep/insomnia

People who have difficulty sleeping may experience various health problems, including memory difficulties.

Stress

Stress is the emotional and physical strain caused by your response to pressure from the outside world. Stress can affect your health in many ways, including memory difficulties.

1.5 Fluctuating abilities and needs

Each person will experience dementia in different ways. There is no definitive direction or path that the condition will follow and there are no exact timescales in which the condition may progress. You have examined how the person's condition will deteriorate over time, but during that time it can also fluctuate or come and go.

Fluctuation of needs and abilities

It is not fully known why somebody with dementia can have 'good days' and 'bad days'. Part of the answer for this could be because we all have good and bad days.

This very much depends on how we are feeling, what we are doing, how much sleep we have had and how we are treated.

When you are having a bad day, everything you do seems to go wrong. Could this be simply because you are feeling so negative? Can your attitude have an effect on the outcome? Think about this for a while. If you do not like doing something, it seems to take forever to get it over and done with. The time drags and your level of boredom or uninterest rises. On the other hand, when you are doing something you enjoy, the time rushes by so that before you know it the activity comes to an end.

This could also apply to the person with dementia. If the person is doing something that is familiar to them, something that they have done many times and have developed a routine for, the person may appear very confident and able to do it with ease. They may appear to show no signs of dementia. However, take the person out of their familiar surroundings and out of their routine, and their confusion will grow, causing their symptoms to be more obvious.

It has been shown that stress has an effect on our memory. In the early stages of dementia, the person may be fully aware that they have forgotten where they have put things. This can cause their stress levels to rise, resulting in added memory difficulties, frustration and confusion. In these earlier stages it is important for you as a care worker to give the person emotional support. Do not be tempted to take over what they are having difficulty with. Help them to calm down and think about what they are doing. The more the person becomes agitated, the greater their difficulties will become.

As the condition progresses, the more support the person will require, including support with day-to-day activities. You can give support by reminding the person what they need to do. Do not overload them, as this will increase their stress and therefore their symptoms. If the person asks you a question and repeats it several times within a short space of time, answer it as though it is the first time you have heard the question. Do not show your frustrations, as this will only cause them to become upset when they see how their behaviour is affecting you.

In the later stages, the person will become emotionally and physically frail. Their reliance on care will increase to the point where they are no longer able to care for themselves. They may lose their ability to eat, walk or speak, perhaps only shouting an occasional word or crying out.

2: Recognising and diagnosing dementia

2.1 The impact of early diagnosis and follow-up to diagnosis

For most people, receiving the diagnosis of dementia is very distressing. It is also very upsetting for their family. Many people today still think of dementia as being a condition that causes people to go 'mad'. It is these negative images that can cause unnecessary distress for both the person and their family.

If you are supporting somebody who is exhibiting any signs or symptoms of forgetfulness, confusion or the inability to find the right words when communicating, it is important that they see their GP. Diagnosis can be difficult to make in the early stages as the symptoms of dementia can develop slowly. They can also be similar to symptoms of other health conditions. The GP or health professional will be able to monitor any pattern of symptoms and undertake tests over a period of time to measure any changes in the person's mental ability. A brain scan can help with diagnosis; this could be a CT scan or MRI scan. If a diagnosis is made, the person may be referred to a specialist for further treatment.

Early diagnosis

The early diagnosis of dementia is essential in order to:

- rule out other conditions that may be treatable
- access advice, information and support
- allow the person with dementia and their family to plan and make arrangements for the future.

Preparing for the future

Receiving an early diagnosis of dementia can help the person and their family to plan and prepare for the future. Although there is no cure at present, there are various medications available which can help improve symptoms and, for some, slow down the progression of the disease. Early diagnosis can help the person to identify and access sources of advice and support for their condition.

The early education of the person and their family can help them to develop a better understanding of what the future may hold. The person will have time to put their finances in order and to make wishes for their funeral through the drawing up of a will. They can be encouraged and supported to sort out any bills and arrange for future bills to be paid by direct debit so that they are not overlooked. The person may find comfort in keeping busy during the initial stages and they may feel reassured that their future has been planned to meet their needs.

Living independently

Following diagnosis, the person may want to live as independently as they can for as long as they can. They may not appreciate someone taking over their life in these early stages when they are still able to care for themselves. To enable the person to remain as independent as possible, encourage them to contact

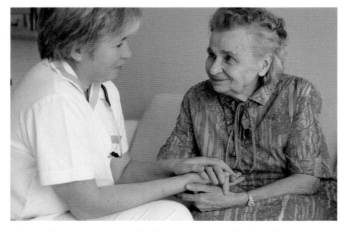

Discussing the future with the person can help with understanding and accepting.

social services, if they have not already done so, to find out what support they could be entitled to. In order to aid their memory, the person could place a list of important telephone numbers by their phone. This way they will always know where a telephone number is if they need it. Labels could be placed on cupboard doors to remind them of the contents. Notes could be placed on doors as a reminder to lock them. Lists could be put on a noticeboard of things to do and days to do them on, such as putting the rubbish out for the refuse collectors.

Continuing with hobbies and interests

The most important thing to support the person with is in continuing to enjoy their life. Support them to continue with their hobbies or interests. One good activity that will help them in the future is the development of a life history book. Encourage and support them to collect together photographs of people who are important to them and events that hold important memories, such as the birth of their first grandchild, their wedding day or family holidays. Encourage the person to label each photograph clearly in the book so that they can look back at it at any time and be reminded of good memories.

Access to specialist services

Early diagnosis can enable the early introduction of specialist services. The services may include:

- family GPs – referring the person for further tests, reviewing medication
- district nurses
- health visitors
- community psychiatric nurses
- consultants
- memory clinics
- neurologists
- geriatricians
- neuropsychiatrists
- physiotherapists
- dieticians
- clinical psychologists
- speech and language therapists.

In many cases, the earlier the diagnosis and follow-up, the sooner the person can start regaining their life again. This is not to say that they will receive a cure – at this moment in time the only option open to people is acceptance and treatment in slowing down the progress of the condition.

2.2 Recording possible signs or symptoms of dementia in line with agreed ways of working

The health and well-being of a person should be monitored on a regular basis to ensure any resulting needs can be actioned without delay. When monitoring somebody's condition, it is important to record any findings in line with your organisation's policies and procedures.

In the very early stages of dementia the person may have days or episodes of forgetfulness which could be put down to the person being off-colour or having an off day. These episodes may be masked by their ability to recall past events easily. They may be able to give a reason as to why they cannot remember what you have just said to them. They may say that the television was too loud and they did not hear you. They may even be adamant that you have not told them anything, giving rise to you questioning your own memory.

The person may have difficulty understanding or following new ideas or regimes. To cover these difficulties they may say that they preferred the old way, as it is not as confusing. They could hide occurrences of misplacing items, making out that someone has moved the item or someone has taken it. All of these events, happenings and reasons could be very genuine and indeed the person themselves may believe that what they are saying is true. If they were all true, the person would be a very unlucky person to be experiencing all of these negative events. The likelihood of them all occurring for the same person in a short space of time would be rather remote.

Misplacing items can be one of the first symptoms of dementia.

Recording all of these occurrences will enable you and the team to build up a picture of the person's mental and physical health. Recording times that they needed reminding to do something or became confused or disorientated will enable you to look back and identify frequencies to ascertain if their memory is deteriorating.

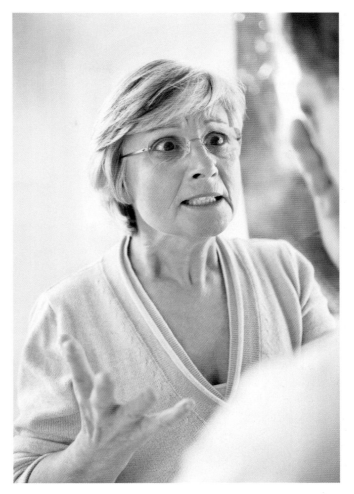

How would you respond if the person you were supporting claimed that you had not told them anything, when you thought that you had?

Involving the family

When supporting somebody with dementia, it may be of immense benefit to involve the family. Encourage and support the family to keep a diary of the person's symptoms. As a care worker, you may not see the person as much as their family do and so they can help to give you a better picture of the person and their needs. The diary that the family compiles could help them and you to identify changes in the person that may be otherwise missed. The diary could also aid in monitoring any current interventions and the resulting benefits to the person.

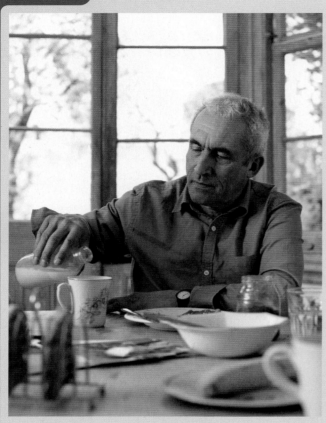

Geoffrey had been living in sheltered housing for a number of years following a stroke. His confidence in his own abilities since the stroke had been very low and he was often heard mumbling to himself. Geoffrey was visited every morning by the warden Leona to check that he was OK. Geoffrey always met Leona on his doorstep as he put out his empty milk bottle. One morning Geoffrey was not on his doorstep as usual, which concerned Leona. She rang his doorbell and waited. Geoffrey came to the door and greeted her with his usual smile. 'Are you all right, Geoff, you haven't put out your empties?' she asked. Geoffrey nodded, scratched his head and replied, 'I'm fine, I haven't finished the bottle yet as I didn't drink much yesterday.' 'As long as you are all right then,' Leona replied, waving goodbye as she turned and walked away.

The following day, once again Geoffrey was not on his doorstep. Leona rang the doorbell again and was greeted by Geoffrey, still wearing the same clothes as he had on the previous day. 'No milk bottles to put out again today?' she asked. Geoffrey agreed, saying he had decided to drink more water: 'I'm cutting down on my cups of tea, getting a bit of a beer belly,' he joked. Leona was a little concerned but then shrugged it off, believing Geoffrey was always getting his words mixed up, due to his age.

As the weeks passed Geoffrey had days when he did not put out any empty bottles, and then he would put out three or four at a time. Some days Geoffrey looked unwashed or unshaven, which was unlike him. Leona was concerned but on talking to Geoffrey she felt she was worrying about nothing. Geoffrey's behaviour had been up and down for over 12 months when Leona announced she was changing her job and a new male warden, Patrick, would be taking over. Geoffrey did not take this news very well and he became agitated, blaming Leona for the death of his wife. Leona was very shocked by this, especially as Geoffrey had never been married. She mentioned this to Patrick during her handover and explained she thought something was not quite right but she could not quite put her finger on it. Patrick asked how long had this been going on for and then said he would take care of it.

1 After visiting each resident in the sheltered housing, what actions should Leona have taken?

2 What concerns would you have had regarding Geoffrey?

3 How would records of Leona's visits to Geoffrey have been of benefit?

4 What actions should Patrick take now regarding Geoffrey?

Suggested monitoring and recording

The person's GP or neurologist may benefit from the information recorded in altering any medications or treatment the person receives. The following areas are those which it is important to monitor and record in the person, as these will show what changes have occurred and over what period:

- memory
- behaviour
- personality
- ability to cope with daily living skills
- care-giving strategies – have they worked?
- activities the person enjoys
- any medications they have taken that day (including prescriptions, over-the-counter and herbal remedies), with details of medication name, dosage, and when and how many taken daily
- what the person has expressed about their abilities and needs.

2.3 Reporting possible signs of dementia

The diagnosis of dementia does not generally occur following the first visit to the GP. Generally there is a process which the person goes through in order to receive a diagnosis. During this process it is vital that you report any potential signs of dementia following your organisation's policies and procedures, and in line with government guidelines.

National Institute for Health and Clinical Excellence (NICE)

The NICE has devised detailed guidelines for supporting people with dementia. These include guidelines to assist with the early diagnosis of dementia. The guide states that primary health care staff should consider referring people who display signs of mild cognitive impairment (MCI) for assessment. The NICE also includes in its guidelines information regarding the diagnosis and assessment of dementia. It states that diagnosis should only be made following comprehensive assessment, which should include:

- the person's history
- a cognitive and mental state examination
- a physical examination
- a review of all medication, including over-the-counter remedies.

Your role in reporting possible signs of dementia

As a care worker, your input in reporting possible signs of dementia would go towards the person's history. Your input can help them receive the care that they need, when they need it. It is for this reason that you should ensure timely reporting of any observations you make or concerns you may have.

To report a concern, you must follow your organisation's guidelines. If you are unsure of what these guidelines are, you should speak with your line manager as soon as possible to ensure your actions follow best practice for the person. In general terms, most reports are given to a designated member of staff. This may be your line manager, supervisor or manager. Your verbal report should be factual and to the point. Try to avoid giving your own opinions. Although opinions can help to look at and clarify various issues from differing viewpoints, they can also be unhelpful if used inappropriately. Once you have given a verbal report, you should back up what you have discussed with the appropriate person, by writing a written report. Again your written report should be factual and detail all of the actions you have taken.

Some reports will have an increased impact if they are delivered in a certain way. For example, you may have been asked to monitor somebody over a set period of time and to report back your findings. Simply writing those findings down may not have the same effect as plotting your findings on a graph. A graph or chart will give a visual representation of your findings, which may give a better explanation as to the person's mental state and any changes that have occurred.

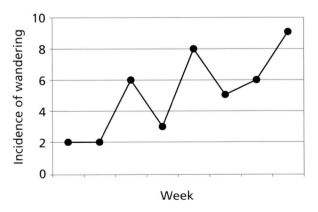

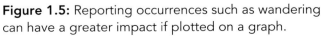

Figure 1.5: Reporting occurrences such as wandering can have a greater impact if plotted on a graph.

Activity 2

Process of reporting

Speak with your line manager or supervisor to identify your organisation's policy and procedures on the process of reporting information.

Functional skills

English: Speaking and listening

The discussion with your manager can be either formal or informal and can give you the opportunity to practise taking part in a one-to-one discussion.

Reflect

Imagine you, or someone you love, have just been given the news that you or they have dementia. Being honest, what would be your initial thoughts or feelings? Do you feel it is OK to feel or think this way? Is there anything you feel that society can do to help with the acceptance and understanding of dementia?

2.4 The impact of a diagnosis of dementia

Receiving news that you know will have a major impact on your future and those who are close to you can be very frightening and overwhelming. The person may feel very insecure at the time, even if they have family and friends around them. The impact on the person and their family and friends can vary; some may see it as a relief that the cause of their difficulties has been diagnosed, while others may be in disbelief, preferring not to acknowledge what they have been told.

Feelings

The person may be shocked on first hearing the diagnosis; this can often turn to denial. One theory on loss or grief shows that the process usually goes through five stages, including:

1 denial

2 anger

3 bargaining

4 depression

5 acceptance.

The person may not necessarily go through each stage in this particular order, and indeed can go backwards and forwards, repeating various stages a number of times before reaching and remaining at acceptance.

The person may experience fear or the concern that they will lose control over their lives and their future. They may also fear becoming a burden on their family and friends. Some may feel guilty, blaming themselves and thinking that they could have prevented their condition from developing.

Whatever feelings the diagnosis creates in the person, you should encourage and support them to talk about their feelings. Some may not feel comfortable voicing their feelings to their family and friends, preferring to talk with someone they do not know. The person's family and friends should not be upset by this decision and should respect the wishes of their loved one.

Initially the person may simply want to curl up and lock out the world around them. Family and friends need to be supportive in these situations. Telling the person to 'get a grip' or that what they are doing is silly is not going to be of any benefit – in fact, it will often make things worse.

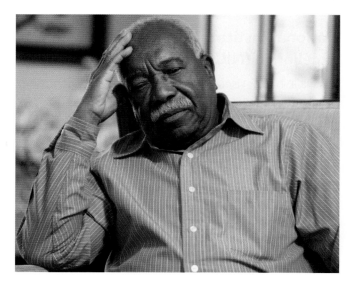

It can take people a long time to reach acceptance in the grief process.

NICE requirements

NICE guidelines state that following a diagnosis of dementia, health and social care professionals should provide the person and their family with written information regarding:

- the signs and symptoms of dementia
- the course and prognosis of the condition
- treatments
- local care and support services

- support groups
- sources of financial and legal advice, and advocacy
- medico-legal issues, including driving
- local information sources, including libraries and voluntary organisations.

Any advice and information given to the person and their family should be recorded in the person's care notes. The confidentiality of the person should be respected if they decide they do not wish any information to be given to their family.

3: Person-centred approaches to dementia care

3.1 Person-centred and non person-centred approaches to dementia care

It is important to remember that people with dementia are individuals first, with their condition of dementia coming second. They may also be mothers, fathers, brothers, sisters, sons or daughters. They may have led a fulfilling life before the condition of dementia took hold of their memories and personality. How could the care of any person be anything other than individual, specific to their needs, involving and respecting their views on how they want their care to be delivered?

Person-centred care is a way of providing care with the person at the centre of everything you do. It is about using life histories to understand their perspective. Another way of describing it is individualised care – care that is given to the person according to their needs, wishes, beliefs and preferences. One would hope that gone are the days when everyone in a care home got up at the same time, ate their breakfast at the same time, got washed and dressed at the same time, even going to the toilet at the same time. These regimented routines of care homes were devised for the benefit of the staff, not the people being supported. The day revolved around tasks and duties that had to be performed, more often than not putting the people's specific needs at the end of the priority list. If you needed support, which type of care home would you choose?

Earlier on in this chapter we looked at how dementia can affect people and identified that no two people will necessarily follow the same process through the condition of dementia. This being the case should automatically prevent all people with dementia being treated in the same way.

Benefits of a person-centred approach

Studies have shown that a person-centred approach can help reduce agitation in the person with dementia. Agitation is often caused by the person's frustration in not being able to express themselves, for example, when they want to express sadness, pain, thirst, hunger or tiredness. Other studies on a person-centred approach have shown that the person often remains living in their own home for longer. A person-centred approach can also ensure that the person does not endure the degrading, discriminatory and abusive practices which could otherwise occur. People and all those involved in their care should feel safe, feel that they are a part of what is going on, receive continuity of care, have purposeful goals which they are supported to progress towards and have a feeling that they do matter.

Case study

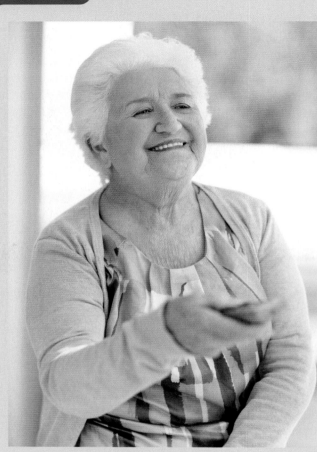

It is approaching lunch time but Mrs Lancaster is not really hungry. She would like a drink and would prefer to remain in her room as she is comfortable and her favourite TV programme is about to start.

Mrs Lancaster is not able to voice these preferences verbally, as she finds it very difficult to verbalise and so has given up trying. Tracy, one of the senior care workers, enters Mrs Lancaster's room and makes her jump, as she did not hear her entering. 'Come on then love, your dinner's ready,' Tracy tells Mrs Lancaster. She then promptly holds Mrs Lancaster under the arm and says, 'Up you come chum.' Mrs Lancaster reels back in pain and cries out. Tracy responds by saying, 'Don't be silly, now come on, your dinner's going to get cold,' again pulling up under Mrs Lancaster's arm. Mrs Lancaster pulls away which makes Tracy annoyed. She bends down and puts her face close to Mrs Lancaster's and says, 'I'll leave you here to starve if you carry on like that.' Mrs Lancaster cannot take any more bullying or threats from Tracy so she brings her head back and then sharply forward, head-butting Tracy. 'You nasty woman, you ought to be locked up doing things like that! What have I ever done to you to deserve treatment like that?' Tracy shouts, leaving the room with a bloodied nose.

1   Explain six things in detail that could have possibly led to Mrs Lancaster head-butting Tracy.

2   What should Tracy have done to prevent this occurrence?

3   Describe a way Mrs Lancaster could be supported to communicate in future.

4   Describe how her care could be given using a person-centred approach.

Identifying needs

As a care worker, you should identify the specific needs of the person with dementia. These needs could arise from their gender, ethnicity, age, religion and personal care. Other needs could also arise from their physical health or physical disability, any sensory impairment, communication difficulties, problems resulting from poor nutrition, poor oral health or learning disabilities. The person's needs should be identified with input from the person, their family, friends and any other people who are important in that person's life.

Once the person's care needs have been identified, plans should be made to draw up a support plan which will describe how those needs will be met, with a real focus on strengths. As with the assessing of needs, the person must be at the centre of the support planning process. Nothing should be planned for them without them.

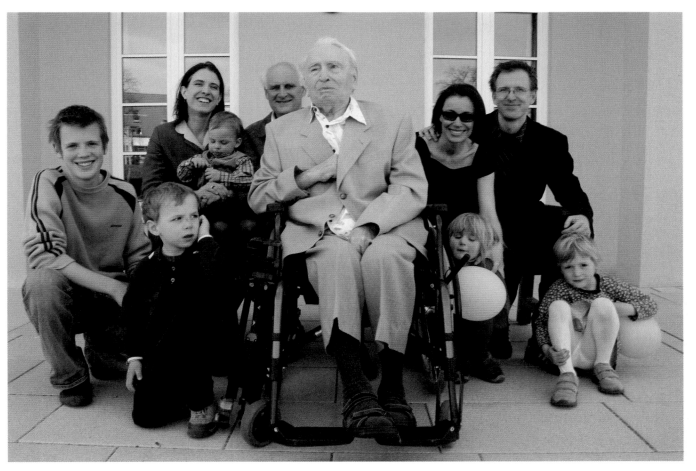

Input from the person's family, friends and relevant others is important to identify the person's needs.

3.2 Different techniques to meet the fluctuating abilities and needs of the individual with dementia

Many people with dementia are able to live in their own homes for most of their lives with care being given to them by their families. It is important that the person is supported to recognise that the condition that they have is not the fault of anyone, especially not their own. When supporting the fluctuating needs and abilities of the person, it is very important that you recognise that they are not responsible for the things that they do. It is not the person who is spitting out their food; it is the condition's effect on the person's ability to communicate which is preventing them from saying, 'I don't like that.' It is not the person who is constantly wandering around the environment; it is the condition that has taken away their spatial awareness.

As a support worker, you must focus on the skills and abilities that the person has, rather than those that they have lost. Ensure that you are fully aware of and respect the person's background, their history and their likes and dislikes. Be prepared for changes and adopt a flexible approach. No two days may be the same in supporting people with dementia. Seize the challenge and look forward to the unexpected. As the saying goes, 'variety is the spice of life'.

Knowing the person

By learning about each person's history and background, you can design the care and support you provide around their specific needs. For example, the person may have been a sergeant major in the army, which could account for them shouting out orders. The person may have experienced a traumatic event in their lives such as being trapped in a collapsed building, which could account for them becoming agitated and screaming when the lights are switched off in their bedroom at night. Without this background knowledge, and more importantly understanding, the person who shouts orders may be wrongly labelled as being noisy and dictatorial. The person who screams in the dark may be wrongly labelled as disruptive and attention-seeking.

A person's physical condition can be affected by their dementia. Their mobility may be reduced, as may their ability to maintain their own personal care or diet. Combining these factors can increase the person's susceptibility to other illnesses such as chest infections or physical conditions such as pressure sores.

Ensure the person's support plan is kept as up to date as possible and shows alternative methods to use for various fluctuations in their support needs. Support other care workers by sharing proven practices. As a support worker, you may have identified triggers to somebody's behaviour. Do not keep this information to yourself; inform other care staff and have it recorded in the person's support plan. The same applies when you identify any new method of supporting the person to meet their fluctuating needs.

Provide a stable environment and suitable surroundings

One of the main triggers that can cause somebody with dementia to become agitated and confused is a change in their routine. Any changes to the person's life or daily routine can cause them to become unsettled, which could lead to inappropriate behaviours. To ensure stability the following factors are important.

- Have consistent, regular staff. Unfamiliar faces can cause the person great upset. Ensure they know the staff and ensure the same staff member provides care to the person in their own home.
- Maintain a familiar environment. In everyone's life it is possible that their surroundings will change at some point. This could simply be through redecoration or changes in furniture. Where possible, if decoration needs to be undertaken within the person's environment, try to make the new decor similar to if not the same as how it was previously. If relocation is required for the person, ensure that the impact is minimised by confirming the suitability of the new location. This will save on the person needing to be relocated again if the environment proves to be unsuitable for their needs.

- Ensure the person is in a non-stressful, constant and familiar environment.
- Establish a regular routine, regular physical activity and adequate exposure to light to improve any sleep disturbances.

Environments can be used positively to enhance memory and reinforce identity. Decorating the environment with things that prompt memory will support orientation and promote well-being. Some environments cause additional confusion because of visual perceptual difficulties. Noisy environments can make people more agitated and affect communication.

Validation

Validation is a technique that is widely practised in the area of dementia care. It is about accepting and supporting the person's feelings, and not persistently challenging their reality. It is about trying to understand the problems that underline the behaviours. It is about showing the person with dementia that you understand the way they are feeling.

Specific strategic support

People with dementia may behave in ways that are completely out of character. Some of these behaviours can be disturbing to onlookers and especially the person's family, when seeing their loved one behaving in a way they have never seen before. The following are examples of the types of behaviours people with dementia may display.

Wandering

People with dementia may tend to walk or 'wander' apparently aimlessly for a variety of reasons. It could be because they are bored or they feel they need to escape or get out of the environment they are in. The person may simply need to use the bathroom but cannot remember where it is. On occasions this wandering may take them out of the house or even down the street. This could lead them to become 'lost' if they are unable to find their way back home. For most people, wandering may only be a short phase that they go through. And, although it is little comfort at the time, people with dementia often retain a good degree of road sense and are seldom involved in traffic accidents. To reduce incidents of wandering, promote physical activities to reduce the person's boredom and to help use some pent-up energy.

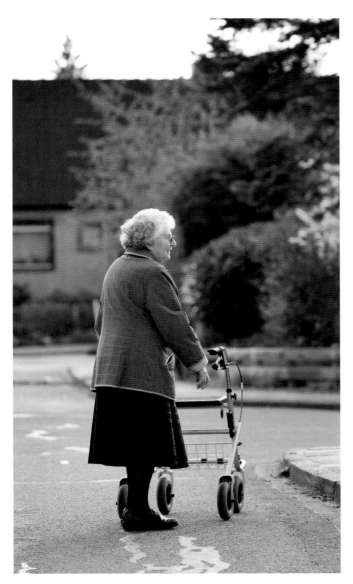

What dangers could wandering have for somebody?

Incontinence

Loss of bowel or bladder control usually occurs as the dementia progresses. Sometimes these accidents may happen because the person cannot remember where the bathroom is or cannot get there in time. If the person does become incontinent, you need to help them to maintain their dignity and respect by being understanding and reassuring. Incontinence pads, sheaths or catheters can be obtained to help keep the person free from unnecessary embarrassment and frustration.

Agitation

Agitation can include behaviours such as sleeplessness, verbal or physical aggression and irritability. These types of behaviour often increase with the stages of dementia and can become quite severe. Agitation may be triggered by a variety of factors, including environmental factors, fear and tiredness. Most often agitation is triggered when the person feels as if they are no longer in control of the situation. You can help reduce episodes of agitation by reducing the intake of caffeine, sugar and processed foods. The reduction of noise or crowds can also help, as does the maintenance of the person's routines.

Repetitive speech or actions

It is common for people who have dementia to repeat a word, statement, question or activity more than once in a short amount of time. This repetition can be frustrating and stressful to the care giver and the person's family. Repetition is often a result of the person becoming anxious, bored, fearful or agitated. One way of reducing this is to provide them with reassurance. Alternative strategies could include displaying reminders of activities around their home such as 'Dinner is at 6:30pm' or 'Dave comes home at 5pm'. This strategy may assist with reducing anxiety and uncertainty about anticipated events.

Paranoia

People with dementia may suddenly become suspicious, jealous or start accusing others of things. When this happens, the person will believe in what they are saying and therefore you should not try to argue or disagree with them. Stay calm and encourage the person to calm down. Ask them what is wrong and let them know that you are there to help them.

Improve your knowledge and understanding

Many organisations have helpful information on understanding and supporting people with dementia. Set yourself a goal to develop your practices through research, talking to people who are in the early stages of dementia or family and friends of those who have it. Learning about dementia from those who have first-hand experience is often more beneficial than reading a book, although books have the benefit of being portable and accessible at any time. At the end of this chapter there is a list for further reading which will help your knowledge and understanding further.

Doing it well

Meeting the needs of people with dementia

- Know the person well, including their history and background.
- Keep their support plan up to date.
- Provide a stable environment and suitable surroundings.
- Ensure specific strategic support.
- Improve your knowledge and understanding.

Dealing with the difficulties that come with the diagnosis of dementia is not going to be made any easier with the myths and stereotypes that society has created. Within society, dementia is often seen as a condition that causes the person to require 24-hour care in a secure environment so they cannot get out and wander aimlessly. People who are newly diagnosed with the condition are sometimes disbelieved because they appear 'normal' and are not dribbling or babbling. Some myths or falsehoods can create an unrealistic hope within the person or their family. Some of these untruths profess to offer cures or preventions. The following information can help you to identify fact from fiction.

> **Q** – *Can using aluminium saucepans affect the risk of developing Alzheimer's?*
>
> **A** – No. There is no convincing evidence that cooking with aluminium saucepans increases the risk of developing Alzheimer's.
>
> **Q** – *Is it true that people who follow a healthy lifestyle reduce the risk of developing dementia?*
>
> **A** – Yes. Research shows that people who enjoy a healthy lifestyle by eating a well-balanced diet, not smoking and taking regular exercise reduce their chances of developing dementia. Recent research has shown that being healthy in mid-life can help lower our risk of developing dementia as we age.
>
> **Q** – *Can Ginkgo Biloba help people with dementia?*
>
> **A** – No. Unfortunately, the latest evidence shows that Ginkgo Biloba has no benefit for people with dementia.
>
> **Q** – *Does eating meat have any connection with developing Alzheimer's?*
>
> **A** – There is no convincing proof that eating meat is linked to developing Alzheimer's.
>
> **Q** – *Do people who have dementia become childlike?*
>
> **A** – No. It is very important to remember that people with dementia are adults and should be treated with the dignity and respect that other adults receive.

3.3 Myths and stereotypes

Many people, quite wrongly, have stereotypes regarding dementia. It is these stereotypes that can become the fear of reality for people newly diagnosed with dementia. Sometimes it is the person's own stereotyping of dementia that they have to face. Facing and resolving this can only occur with education and acceptance.

Activity 3

What's in a name?

Devise a simple questionnaire which you can either give to colleagues within your organisation, or to your family and friends. Ask questions such as, 'Give the first word that comes into your head when you hear the word "dementia".' Include a few questions that relate to the myths around dementia to see if your colleagues or family know the truth or not. Compile the results from your questionnaire and discuss these with your assessor.

People's inappropriate views or opinions on dementia often arise from ignorance. For many, the only portrayal they have of dementia is that which they see on television. Storylines shown in films are often of people in the advanced stages of dementia. If this is the only perspective you have, then there is no wonder why society looks at this condition in the way it does. If the individual newly diagnosed with dementia or their family has only ever known of dementia in this way, then their fears will understandably be heightened.

3.4 Overcoming fears

Research has shown that many people fear the thought of developing a form of dementia. The worry of losing one's identity, independence and mind for some is a greater fear than the fear of death. Worrying about a condition that you may not develop seems futile. Worrying about a condition that you have developed will not do your health much good.

Simply telling somebody who has received a diagnosis of dementia or their family not to worry is insufficient. Advising the person and their family to talk about their fears will help towards them overcoming any uncertainties. Ignoring the condition or pretending it is not happening is simply denial. To help all those involved to overcome worries about the future, the person and their family should be supported to learn the truth, what they can expect from the future.

Understand the condition

The person and their family should be supported to develop a true understanding of the condition they are facing. Information can be obtained from GPs' surgeries, health centres, libraries and the Internet. When obtaining information from books or the Internet, you need to ensure it is up to date and reliable. Internet sites for organisations such as the Alzheimer's Society and NHS Direct can be seen as reliable sites, as can educational sites such as those ending with .org. Some of the facts relating to dementia do not always make for easy reading; however, the person and family need to know what to expect. Information should be provided sensitively and in a format that is accessible to the person and their carers.

Encourage future planning

Once the person and their family are aware of how dementia may affect the future, they should be supported to think ahead and be ready for the changes that will follow. The person and their family will need to prepare things not just materially but emotionally as well. At some point the person may require support with toileting and other personal care needs. They may not want their family attending to this sort of personal care, preferring to have a care worker attend to their needs at home. There may come a point when the person is unable to stay in their own home due to the advancement of their condition. The fear of this eventuality can create a lot of worry for them. Supporting the person to plan for this can help allay those fears. The person may want to use the provisions of the Mental Capacity Act 2005 to make some advanced decisions. They and their family could be supported to identify a care home which the person may move

into in the future. Simply knowing that this step has been arranged can help them feel a little easier, knowing that they will not be placing a burden on their family.

Making life easier

The person may have received a diagnosis of dementia because of their current memory difficulties. The family may worry that the person will not be able to cope very well at home, forgetting to take their medication, forgetting to lock doors and windows when going out and so on. These sorts of worries for the family will not necessarily lessen. As each day passes they may worry. As each day passes the person's condition may increase, making the family worry all the more until it becomes a vicious circle. To help reduce these fears, the person can be supported to remain as independent as possible at home with the use of notes, labels, lists – any memory joggers. The environment in which the person lives can be made safer – for example, installing grab rails or an emergency pull cord system. Making these minor changes to the person's home may reduce the natural worries of the family with regard to their loved one's safety.

Dealing with the diagnosis of dementia is never going to be easy. Some people and their families may benefit from receiving counselling. This can often be provided by the GP's surgery. It is a confidential service which is there to help the person and their family to develop ways of dealing with their thoughts, fears and feelings.

Reflect

Think about the support you have offered people and their families to overcome their fears. Was it appropriate? Did it benefit the person and their family? Is there anything else you now feel you should have done or said differently?

Getting ready for assessment

You need to be able to demonstrate that you have the knowledge for each of the assessment criteria listed in the standards. You can demonstrate your knowledge with written or verbal explanations. This can be achieved by answering questions, either in written form or verbally, which have been set by your assessor. Your knowledge can also be demonstrated using case studies or professional discussions.

You may wish to undertake a written research project covering as many of the assessment criteria as possible. Your project could include real-life case studies where you have examined what effects dementia has had on the people you work with. When using real-life case studies, you must be mindful of confidentiality and seek permission from the appropriate person. This could be your manager or a relative of the person concerned.

You may want to arrange to talk to relatives of people who have dementia; again, you will need to seek the support of your manager before doing this. Talking to relatives would be of benefit for outcomes 1.2, 2.1, 2.4, 3.3 and 3.4. When talking to relatives, you will need to be sensitive to their feelings, especially if the person has been diagnosed recently.

This unit does not have any requirements for observations.

Further reading and research

- www.alzheimers.org.uk (Alzheimer's Society: the UK's leading care and research charity for people with dementia and those who care for them. The organisation provides information, support, guidance and referrals to other appropriate organisations).
- www.bild.org.uk (British Institute of Learning Disabilities: an organisation that works to improve the lives of people with disabilities. It provides a range of published and online information).
- www.cjdsupport.net (an organisation that supports people with prion diseases, including forms of Creutzfeldt-Jakob disease (CJD). It provides a range of information on the various forms of prion disease, and works with professionals to improve the level of care provided for people with these conditions).
- www.hda.org.uk (Huntington's Disease Association: provides information, advice, support and useful publications for families affected by Huntington's disease in England and Wales. It can put you in touch with a regional adviser and your nearest branch or support group).
- Dementia – A NICE–SCIE Guideline on supporting people with dementia and their carers in health and social care – National Clinical Practice Guideline Number 42 (available as a PDF download from http://guidance.nice.org.uk/CG42).

Understand the administration of medication to individuals with dementia using a person-centred approach

The safe administration of medications is vital for all people, but it is of particular importance for people with dementia. Regarding medication, many professionals find it difficult to balance choice and control with risk. In order to give people choice over their lives, it is important that people are given every possible support in order to manage their own medication.

It is surprising what can be achieved with the right support – and the right attitudes. Of course, it must be clear that people manage their own medication safely and without putting themselves or others at serious risk of harm.

Currently medication does not cure dementia but manages the symptoms, improving people's quality of life. Medication has also long been used to sedate people with dementia. The use of antipsychotic drugs has recently been the subject of extensive review, and the position of all UK governments is to promote a reduction in the use of antipsychotic medication.

When you have completed this unit you will:

- understand the common medications for people with dementia
- understand how to provide person-centred care through effective use of medication.

1: Common medications for people with dementia

1.1 Medications used to treat symptoms of dementia

All medicines are regulated through various Acts of Parliament and regulations. They are split into classifications by the Medicines Act 1968.

The Medicines Act covers all substances which are used as medicinal products or ingredients in medicinal products. This Act divides medicines into three categories:

1 Prescription-only medicine (POM). These are medicines that are prescribed for a patient and subsequently supplied by a pharmacist. These medicines can only be obtained with a prescription from a GP, a dentist, a vet or another person who is qualified to prescribe. This includes midwives and nurses who have achieved the qualifications to be a Non-Medical Prescriber. They include the medicines that are used to treat the symptoms of dementia. All controlled drugs are prescription only – see below for information about the special requirements for controlled drugs.

2 Over-the-counter (OTC) or Pharmacy Medicine (P). This type of medicine is supplied by a pharmacist but can be dispensed without a prescription. However, these medicines are sold under the 'supervision' of a pharmacist. Over-the-counter or pharmacy medicines include such items as very strong painkillers, some forms of cold or flu remedies and a wide range of specialist preparations that are designed to alleviate the symptoms of common illnesses. The list of these medicines has increased considerably in recent years and now includes 'morning after' contraception in some areas.

3 General sales list (GSL). These are medicines that need not be obtained through a pharmacist and are freely available in shops and supermarkets. They include mild painkillers and preparations designed to cause temporary alleviation of symptoms of some mild common illnesses, such as throat lozenges and those designed to clear congestion.

Pharmacy stamp	Age	Title, Forename, Surname & Address
	D.o.B	
Try not to stamp over age box		
Number of days' treatment N.B. Ensure dose is stated		NHS Number:
Endorsements		

- A prescription is valid for 13 weeks from the date it was written.
- The only exception is a prescription for controlled drugs, which is valid for only 28 days from the date of issue.
- The name and address of the doctor must be stamped on the prescription.
- Prescriptions can be computer written or hand written, but must be signed by the doctor or other registered clinician to be valid.

Signature of Prescriber   Date

For dispenser No. of Prescns. on form

NHS   PATIENTS – please read the notes overleaf

Figure 2.1: An example of a prescription form

In hospital, residential care or nursing home settings all drugs are kept in lockable cupboards. Where people are self-medicating, they will have a lockable cupboard in their room in which to keep medicines. Fridges and even portable drugs trolleys need to be lockable. Naturally, in someone's own home, it is not necessary to keep drugs in locked containers or cupboards but they should, wherever possible, be kept in a secure cupboard, and must be kept out of the reach of children.

When a pharmacist supplies prescription drugs they must be labelled. The label must show:

- the name of the patient
- the date of the prescription
- the name of the drug
- the quantity in the container
- the dosage to be taken
- any specific instructions about how to take the medication
- the name of the pharmacist supplying the medication.

If the drugs are supplied for someone who is in hospital, the label is also likely to show their unit number, their date of birth and the name of their consultant.

Controlled drugs (CDs)

These are powerful medicines that are usually prescribed for serious conditions and pain relief. They are subject to abuse when taken without a medical reason. They include drugs such as diamorphine, fentanyl and methylphenidate. There are additional safety precautions and requirements for their storage, administration, records and disposal, which are laid down in the Misuse of Drugs Regulations 2001.

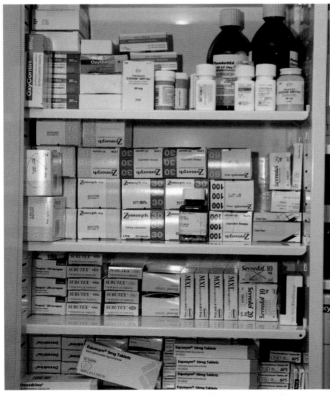

Do you know about the requirements for storage of controlled drugs?

These drugs are very powerful and, although they are very beneficial to the people for whom they are prescribed, they are open to being misused. The additional precautions are necessary, not only because they are highly dangerous if given to the wrong person or in the wrong dosage, but also because many controlled drugs are valuable to criminals who supply illegal drugs.

The requirements for residential care settings do not apply if people are being supported in their own home. The requirements for controlled drugs in residential provision are as follows.

- Secure storage is required for controlled drugs.
- Hard bound registers are recommended for controlled drugs record keeping.
- It is recommended good practice that there is a second member of staff as a witness when CDs are administered.
- Special arrangements must be made for the disposal of controlled drugs.

Activity 1

Copy and complete the table with at least two examples of drugs from each classification:

Prescription-only medicine (POM)	
Over-the-counter/pharmacy OTC/P	
General sales list (GSL)	

Drugs for dementia

People are prescribed medication for many reasons; someone with dementia may also need medication for conditions such as arthritis, diabetes and high blood pressure. However, there are medications that are useful for treating some of the symptoms of dementia. These medications are not able to cure dementia, but they can slow down the progression of symptoms and reduce some of the distress caused by confusion and disorientation.

Medication should never be a first response; it is always better to look for other ways of supporting people wherever possible. For example, if someone is distressed because they are unsure of where they are, providing reassurance and clear and simple signs and reminders can go a long way towards improving people's lives. Medication may then be avoided or reduced.

The current NICE guidelines only recommend drug treatment for the symptoms of two forms of dementia: Alzheimer's disease and dementia with Lewy Bodies. This section does not cover antipsychotic medication – this type of medication is a very important issue in relation to dementia and is covered in section 1.3 below.

The most common drugs used for treating the symptoms of dementia fall into two groups that act in different ways to reduce dementia symptoms. They both act on enzymes in the brain and so have an effect on the neurotransmitters and slow down the progression of symptoms. You are likely to come across the generic and the proprietary or brand names for these drugs, which are listed in Table 2.1.

Table 2.1: Medicines used to treat the symptoms of dementia

Generic name	Proprietary/Brand name
Donepezil hydrochloride	Aricept
Galantamine	Reminyl
Rivastigmine	Exelon
Memantine	Exiba

People with dementia can develop conditions such as depression, anxiety and sleep disturbance. Bearing in mind that medication should never be the first option, sometimes it can prove helpful for people to be prescribed medicines to relieve a condition and improve their quality of life. Commonly used medicines for depression are listed in Table 2.2.

Table 2.2: Medicines used to treat depression

Generic name	Proprietary/Brand names
Fluoxetine	Prozac, Sarafem, Fontex
Parexotine	Seroxat, Aropax, Paxil
Fluvoxamine	Luvox
Citalopram	Cipramil, Celexa
Amitriptyline	Tryptizol, Elavil, Laroxyl, Sarotex
Imipramine	Tofranil, Antideprin, Depsol, Eupramin

Sleep disturbance is common in people with dementia, although it is important that people are supported to follow their own sleep routines. Older people will, in any case, sleep less than younger people, and it may suit some people to sleep for shorter periods spread throughout a full day. Sometimes, a lifestyle change can help with sleep disturbance, for example, if someone starts taking more exercise and being more active during the day, they may be more ready for sleep at night. Rest and sleep are important, but it may not be important that it takes place at the time that you think it should.

The medicines used to treat sleep disturbance are known as hypnotic medicines. Commonly prescribed hypnotic medicines are listed in Table 2.3.

Table 2.3: Medicines used to treat sleep disturbance

Generic name	Proprietary/Brand name
Zopiclone	Zimovane
Zolpidem	Stilnoct
Nitrazepam	Mogadon
Flurazepam	Dalmane

Anxiety is another common condition that can develop as a symptom of dementia. Again, medication should be a last resort – reassurance and support should be the first response when someone becomes anxious and distressed. However, if medication does prove to be necessary, then benzodiazepines are the group of drugs most likely to be prescribed. The most common ones are listed in Table 2.4.

Table 2.4: Medicines used to treat anxiety

Generic name	Proprietary/Brand name
Diazepam	Valium
Lorazapam	Ativan
Alprazolam	Xanax

Activity 2

Check the medications prescribed for the people you support. See how many are on the lists in Tables 2.1–2.4. If there are any that are not included, find out what they are and what they are used for. Make sure you understand what medication people are taking and why they are taking it.

1.2 Effects of medications

All medications cause changes in the body; some of these are beneficial and others are not. Medicines used to treat dementia do have side effects and, as with all medicines, the benefits have to be weighed against the side effects.

If it has not been possible to improve the symptoms of dementia sufficiently using non-medical support, then a prescribed medicine may be helpful for some people.

Dementia medication

Memantine is a dementia drug that has been studied since the early 21st century. It appears to have beneficial effects on slowing down memory loss and in helping people to continue to function in their daily lives. It also appears to reduce aggressive behaviour and makes people calmer and less agitated. This drug is the subject of further studies, but it does not seem to have many unpleasant side effects.

Other anti-dementia drugs such as donepezil and galantamine are known to delay the onset of some of the symptoms of dementia, although they are not usually used after the onset of symptoms because there is little evidence that they improve symptoms which are already present.

Antidepressants

Where people have behavioural conditions such as depression, erratic moods, irritability or verbal aggression, then antidepressants may help to improve their mood and to stabilise mood swings. There are two different types of anti-depressants.

Tricyclic antidepressants have been around for a long time. These include amitriptyline and imipramine. Generally these are not recommended for people with dementia as there appears to be some evidence that they may increase confusion. They also cause dizziness as a common side effect, which is clearly risky for older people if they are prone to falls.

Selective serotonin re-uptake inhibitors (SSRIs) are a newer form of antidepressants and they work in a different way. They include fluoxetine and parexotine. Trials and studies have shown that these are more effective for older people with dementia and have fewer side effects. Occasionally people may feel nauseous when they start to take them, but this usually subsides after a few weeks.

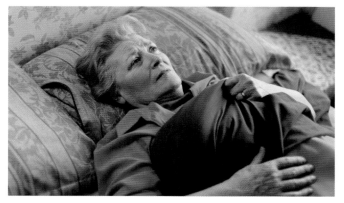

Sleep disturbance can have a great impact on a person's mental functioning.

Sleep disturbance

Disturbed sleeping patterns can be a symptom of dementia, involving wakefulness or restless wandering. If it is determined that medication is necessary, hypnotic drugs may be prescribed to make people sleep. These work by providing sedation in order to get someone off to sleep.

One of the problems is that many of the traditional hypnotic drugs can leave people still feeling sedated the next day or, if the person does wake during the night, they are more likely to be confused, disorientated and possibly unsteady because of the sedation. Clearly, this can be a major risk, particularly if people are in their own homes without carer support.

Anxiety medication

Usually, anxiety in people with dementia can be improved by providing support and reassurance, but serious anxiety coupled with panic attacks may require some medication. Frequently, anxiety states will improve through the use of anti-depressants. Sometimes, benzodiazepines will be prescribed, although there are risks of excessive sedation for people with dementia. Excessive sedation can result in increased confusion and unsteadiness and can also reduce memory function. So although it reduces the anxiety, this type of medication may increase some of the symptoms of dementia.

> **Reflect**
>
> Think about the medications used in your workplace. Do you think that medication is sometimes used for the convenience of the staff so that people are quiet and calm in the day and sleep during the night? Although it may be difficult to have people wandering around, can you see how medication can deprive people of rights and choices about their lives?

1.3 Antipsychotic medication

Antipsychotic medication is used to treat **psychosis**. When someone is experiencing a psychotic episode they are unable to tell the difference between reality and what is in their imagination. Some people experience **hallucinations** where they will see things that are not really there, but they are very real to the person concerned. They may also experience **delusions** where they believe things that are not true; again, they are very real to the person concerned.

Antipsychotic drugs were first used in the 1950s and 1960s. They were developed for people who experienced psychotic symptoms as the result of serious conditions such as schizophrenia or bipolar disorder. While they help to improve psychotic conditions, they do have significant side effects, including over-sedation, rigidity of movement and tremors (similar to Parkinson's disease), involuntary chewing movements, low blood pressure and mobility problems.

In the past 20 years different types of antipsychotic drugs have been developed that have fewer side effects. However, there is little evidence that these medications actually benefit people with dementia. A major government report in 2009 ('The use of antipsychotic medication for people with dementia: Time for Action', Professor Sube Banerjee) identified that about 180,000 people with dementia were being prescribed antipsychotic drugs. The report estimated that as few as 20 per cent (36,000) of these people were likely to be getting any benefit from them. The report also identified that an additional 1,800 deaths and 1,620 strokes were happening as a result of the use of antipsychotics and the adverse reactions they caused.

The most commonly used antipsychotic drugs are listed in Table 2.5.

Table 2.5: Common antipsychotic drugs

Generic name	Proprietary/brand name
Chlorpromazine	Largactil
Fluphenazine	Modecate
Haloperidol	Serenace, Haldol
Risperidone	Risperdal
Trifluoperazine	Stelazine
Amisulpride	Solian

The National Institute for Health and Clinical Excellence (NICE) has issued guidelines for the use of antipsychotics. It advises that the use of these drugs is always a last resort and should only be considered where all other interventions have failed. The criteria for prescribing and administering antipsychotic drugs to people with dementia are that they should only be prescribed for those with severe symptoms. NICE guidelines do not recommend the use of antipsychotic drugs for anyone experiencing mild to moderate symptoms.

> **Key terms**
>
> **Psychosis** – an episode when someone is out of touch with reality.
> **Hallucinations** – seeing things that are not really there.
> **Delusions** – believing things that are not real.

One of the problems with using antipsychotic drugs is that there is no evidence that the hallucinations, delusions and challenging behaviour shown by people with dementia are caused in the same way as those experienced by people with serious mental health conditions such as schizophrenia or bipolar disorder.

The use of such medication in residential and nursing homes has raised particular concerns. These medications are often called the 'chemical cosh' because the sedative effects of the drugs can make it easier for staff to manage the behaviour of people who present challenges. The guidelines are clear that medication can only be used for the benefit of the individual with dementia and not for the benefit of the management of the home. All of the inspectorates in the UK now check that residential and nursing homes are complying with the NICE guidelines regarding the use of antipsychotic drugs. It is also clear under the Mental Capacity Act and the Deprivation of Liberty Safeguards that if someone is prevented from leaving a residential or nursing home through the use of medication to sedate them, they may be deprived of their liberty and there should be an appropriate assessment undertaken.

> **Activity 3**
>
> Check on the use of antipsychotic drugs in your workplace. Find out how widely they are used and the reasons why they are prescribed for particular individuals. Make notes about the most common drugs prescribed, then research information about the drugs, their side effects and the guidelines that cover their use.

Case study

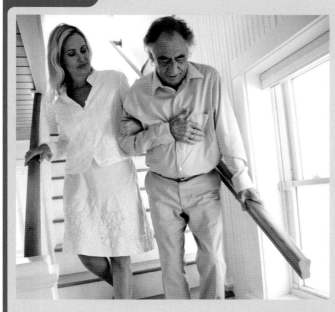

Jim is 83 and has Alzheimer's disease. Following the death of his wife, his symptoms became more obvious. At first, he managed at home with daily visits from his daughter, Christine, but as he became more anxious and disturbed at night and began to go out of the house, he came to live with his daughter. Generally Jim copes well; he does ask repeated questions and tends to get lost if he goes to the local shops on his own, but he enjoys doing the garden and grows all the vegetables for the family. He does get up during the night and becomes agitated because he cannot find his wife, but Christine offers him reassurance and he returns to bed.

Christine arranged a respite bed for three weeks in a local residential home so that she and her husband could have a break, but when she visited her father in the residential home she found him sitting in an armchair, looking sleepy and confused. His head was on one side and he was making chewing movements and 'pulling faces'. His movements were very slow and when he got up he was shuffling along. When she asked what had happened she was told that this was just normal deterioration of his condition. On being handed his medicines, she noticed some new ones. The staff explained that he was so disruptive and wandering at night they had asked the home's GP to prescribe antipsychotics to 'calm him down'. Christine was very concerned and felt that the medication had had a very negative effect on her father.

Case study

Hyacinth is 78; she has Alzheimer's disease and lives in extra care housing. Over the past six months she has had increasing episodes of hallucinations, which can occur at any time of the day. These cause her to become very distressed and terrified as she believes that creatures are going to harm her. During these episodes, she begins screaming and cowering in corners; she is very frightened and takes several hours to calm down. She is then fearful and unsettled almost continually.

Following discussions with the team working to support Hyacinth, it was decided to try her on risperidone for a short period to see if this would improve her symptoms and make her less distressed. After a week on the medication, support staff noticed a definite improvement. Hyacinth was much less distressed, she had no hallucinations and, although she was still confused and very forgetful, she was not constantly frightened and was much calmer.

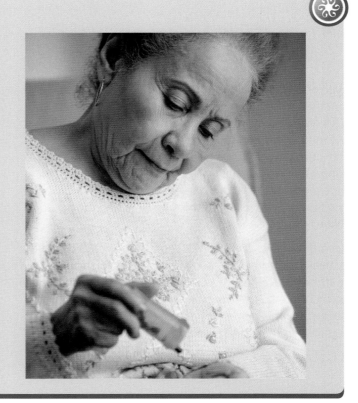

Activity 4

Read the two case studies about Jim and Hyacinth. Make notes on the points for and against the use of antipsychotics presented in these two situations.

Think of another situation, perhaps involving someone you support, and make notes for and against the use of antipsychotics in that situation.

Reflect

Do you think that there are times in your workplace when medication has been used for the convenience of staff? Are there times when medication has been used for the benefit of other residents because of the effects of someone's behaviour? Do you think this is the right thing to do?

Whose rights should take priority?
- the individual with severe symptoms
- the majority of residents
- the staff who have to be able to provide support to everyone.

Think about these issues and discuss them with colleagues if possible.

1.4 Recording and reporting side effects/adverse reactions

Everyone who is being supported to take medication, whether in their own home or in residential care, will have a Medical Administration Record (MAR) chart. This shows the medication prescribed for the person, the dose and the times that it is to be taken. It also shows when a new supply of medicine has arrived. It is used to record each time medicine is taken, as well as any adverse drug reactions (ADRs) to any of the medicines and the action taken in response.

Recording ADRs on the MAR chart is important because it means that other staff or carers will be able to see that there have been problems and the reactions can be monitored. ADRs must also be reported to the doctor who prescribed the medicine so that they can be recorded in the patient's records.

It is also important that the person's views and feelings about their medication are checked and recorded. They should be encouraged to self-report any symptoms they

have and you should ensure that there is a process in place to check each day and record their views.

The pharmacist who dispensed the medicine also needs to know because they will maintain records of ADRs and they may see a trend of adverse reactions to a particular medication or in people who are taking a particular combination of medicines. Pharmacists are often in a better position than individual GPs to notice if there are significant numbers of people reacting to a particular drug or combination of drugs because they deal with far larger numbers than a single GP does. A pharmacy will dispense medicines for several GP practices in an area.

What are side effects and adverse drug reactions?

Side effects are usually the known and expected, although unwanted, consequences of taking a particular medicine. The term 'adverse drug reaction' (ADR) means the same as side effect, but is often used to describe sudden, violent and serious reactions to taking a drug. The term ADR tends to be used only by health and care professionals. The general public are more likely to use the term 'side effects' to cover any reaction to medications.

The side effects of a medicine may be unpleasant, such as nausea, or undesirable, such as drowsiness, but they are not usually serious or harmful for most people. However, as we have seen with the possible effects

---

PATIENT INFORMATION LEAFLET

> **Donepezil hydrochloride 5 mg Tablets**
> **Donepezil hydrochloride 10 mg Tablets**

Read all of this leaflet carefully before you start taking this medicine.
- Keep this leaflet. You may need to read it again.
- If you are a caregiver and will be giving Donepezil hydrochloride to the person you look after, it is also important that you read this leaflet on their behalf.
- If you have any further questions, ask your doctor or pharmacist.
- This medicine has been prescribed for you. Do not pass it on to others. It may harm them, even if their symptoms are the same as yours.
- If any of the side effects become serious, or if you notice any side effects not listed in this leaflet, please tell your doctor or pharmacist.

IN THIS LEAFLET YOU WILL FIND:
1. What Donepezil hydrochloride is and what it is used for
2. Before you take Donepezil hydrochloride
3. How to take Donepezil hydrochloride
4. Possible side effects
5. How to store Donepezil hydrochloride
6. Further information

Can you think of any patient information leaflets you have referred to recently?

of antipsychotics on people with dementia, the side effects can sometimes cause serious problems. In such circumstances decisions have to be made that weigh the benefits of the drug against the potential side effects.

Possible side effects are usually identified during drug trials and people are warned about them in the patient information leaflet (PIL) that must be included with all medicines.

Looking out for side effects

Not all medications suit everyone and some may cause sudden or serious adverse reactions in some people. You must be alert to the possibility of an adverse reaction and ensure that it is reported immediately and emergency medical attention obtained if necessary. When someone has had an adverse drug reaction, it is important that they are monitored closely to ensure that there are no ongoing health issues.

ADRs can take various forms, so it is important to be alert for anything unusual. Common ADRs may include:

- breathing difficulties
- swelling of the face or mouth
- nausea
- vomiting
- sudden rashes or blotches
- confusion
- hallucinations or delusions.

Not all ADRs are so dramatic or so sudden. You may notice some of them over a period of time. Some ADRS may not become evident until a large amount of data has been collected. For example, it was many years before the link was established between certain types of contraceptive pill and an increased risk of blood clots.

Recording and reporting

The recording and reporting of ADRs is important on more than one level. It is important for:

- the individual concerned
- the person who prescribed the medication
- the person who dispensed the medication
- the agencies that regulate medications
- the company that makes and supplies the medication.

The Medicines and Healthcare products Regulatory Agency (MHRA) is responsible for regulating medicines in the UK. It operates a national reporting system so that information on serious side effects or ADRs can be collected and monitored. In this way, the MHRA can identify if a particular medicine has serious side effects. Some medicines have been withdrawn as a result of the information gathered about harmful side effects; others have had their licence restricted to use in certain circumstances only.

In addition to recording any adverse drug reactions on the person's MAR chart and informing the prescribing doctor and dispensing pharmacist, in certain circumstances you also need to report them to the MHRA. ADRs must be reported to the MHRA if the reaction:

- is serious – fatal or life threatening, or resulting in hospitalisation
- is the result of a new medication
- occurs in children.

ADRs should be reported to the MHRA using the Yellow Card Scheme. The MHRA has a standard card that is used to record all the necessary information about an adverse reaction. This reporting enables the MHRA to gather widespread information on medications. The easiest way to make the report is online using the Yellow Card website www.yellowcard.gov.uk. There is also a form that can be completed and sent by post.

Activity 5

Find out about the reporting system in your workplace. Check on information recorded on the MAR charts and see if it covers all the necessary information. Find out who is responsible for reporting ADRs in your workplace.

Look at the website for the Yellow Card Scheme. Download a blank form and practise completing it. DO NOT send it off, but keep a copy so that you have a reference document if you do need to report an ADR.

1.5 PRN medication for people with dementia

Pro re nata is a Latin term that means 'as the circumstance arises' or 'as needed'. In medicine this term has been shortened to PRN and is used to describe medicine that is not taken on a regular basis but is used as and when it is required. This is the usual way of prescribing medication such as pain relief, indigestion remedies, anti-anxiety medication or laxatives.

SUSPECTED ADVERSE DRUG REACTIONS

If you suspect an adverse reaction may be related to one or more drugs/vaccines/complementary remedies, please complete this Yellow Card. See 'Adverse reactions to drugs' section in BNF or www.mhra.gov.uk yellowcard for guidance. Do not be put off reporting because some details are not known.

PATIENT DETAILS

Patient initials   Sex: M / F   Ethnicity   Weight if known (kg)
Age (at time of reaction):
          Identification number (e.g. your practice or hospital ref):

SUSPECTED DRUG(S)/VACCINE(S)

Drug/Vaccine (Brand if known)	Batch Route Dosage	Date started	Date stopped	Prescribed for

SUSPECTED REACTION Please describe the reaction(s) and any treatment given

Date reaction(s) started: Date reaction(s) stopped:
Do you consider the reactions to be serious? Yes / No
If yes, please indicate why the reaction is considered to be serious (please tick all that apply):

Patient died due to reaction	Involved or prolonged inpatient hospitalisation
Life threatening	Involved persistent or significant disability or incapacity
Congenital abnormality	Medically significant; please give details:

OTHER DRUG(S) (including self-medication and complementary remedies)

Did the patient take any other medicines/vaccines/complementary remedies in the last 3 months prior to the reaction? Yes / No
If yes, please give the following information if known:

Drug/Vaccine (Brand if known)	Batch Route Dosage	Date started	Date stopped	Prescribed for

Additional relevant information e.g. medical history, test results, known allergies, rechallenge (if performed), suspect drug interactions. For congenital abnormalities please state all other drugs taken during pregnancy and the last menstrual period.

Please list any medicines obtained from the internet:

REPORTER DETAILS	**CLINICIAN (if not the reporter)**
Name and professional address:	Name and professional address:
Postcode: Tel No:	Postcode: Tel No:
Email:	Email:
Speciality:	Speciality:
Signature: Date:	Date:

Information on adverse drug reactions received by the MHRA can be downloaded at **www.mhra.gov.uk/daps**. Stay up to date on the latest advice for the safe use of medicines with our monthly bulletin Drug Safety Update at **www.mhra.gov.uk/drugsafetyupdate**

Figure 2.2: Have you used the Yellow Card Scheme before?

Pain relief for people with dementia is an area of concern. There is evidence from several studies that pain relief is not provided in the same way as it is to people who do not have dementia. For example, a study of people following hip replacement surgery found that people with dementia received less than half the pain relief of people without dementia.

There are many reasons why people feel pain, particularly as they grow older. Joints are less supple and become stiff and painful; people may develop arthritis; digestive systems may not work as well through lack of exercise and people may have indigestion, constipation or urinary tract infections.

Recognising symptoms of pain

There are many people working in both health and social care who fail to recognise when people with dementia are in pain. There is also a view held by some that people with dementia do not feel pain in the same way as people without dementia. There is absolutely no evidence to support this view and it is vital that all those who support people with dementia are clear that not understanding pain is not the same as not feeling it.

It is essential that you are aware of the possibility that someone may be in pain. People with severe dementia symptoms may not be able to say how they feel; they may not even be able to understand the pain that they are feeling or recognise what it is. That does not mean that they are not in pain, and it certainly does not mean that they should not be provided with pain relief.

Do not forget that all behaviour is a form of communication and it may be that someone's constant pleas to be helped or moaning aloud is an expression of pain rather than simply 'challenging behaviour'.

Look out for other signs of pain rather than relying on someone to tell you. A tool (Abbey pain tool, www.dementiacareaustralia.com) that is used to help to identify pain and discomfort in people with dementia identifies six possible signs of pain:

1 making sounds: whimpering, groaning, crying
2 facial expressions: looking tense, frowning, grimacing, looking frightened
3 changes in body language: fidgeting, rocking, guarding part of body, withdrawn
4 behavioural changes: increased confusion, refusing to eat, alteration in usual patterns

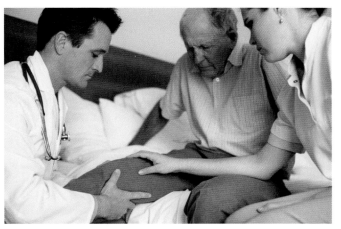

How would you find out where this person was feeling pain?

5 bodily changes: raised temperature, pulse rate or blood pressure, perspiring, flushing or looking very pale
6 physical changes: skin tears, pressure areas, arthritis, contractures, previous injuries.

Any one of these could be an indication that someone is suffering. The best way to find out if someone is in pain is of course to ask them. Keep your questions simple and closed: 'Does it hurt?' 'Is it sore?' Try pointing to part of their body, or your own, if you suspect where the pain may be.

Administering PRN medication

PRN medication should be available for people as and when they need it. Most people will be prescribed paracetamol or maybe stronger codeine-based pain relief. These medicines will need to be kept in the drugs cupboard or with the person's medicines if they are self-medicating. You will need to ensure that people can access pain relief when they need it; they should not have to wait for a medicines round or for when it is convenient for the staff. The point of PRN medication is that it should be used when it is needed.

Activity 6

Think about the people you support. Are you sure that you have not misunderstood some behaviour that was really telling you that someone was in pain? Think about the signs and create a checklist so that you always check people's behaviour in future to ensure that pain is not the reason for agitation or behaviour that challenges.

2: Person-centred care and medication

2.1 Person-centred ways of administering medicines

The administration of medicine is one of the three areas of responsibility. All medicines must be:

- prescribed
- dispensed
- administered.

Prescribing

Usually, the person's general practitioner (GP) will prescribe their medicines, but medicines can sometimes be prescribed by others, such as a hospital consultant, dentist or a qualified midwife or nurse prescriber.

The person prescribing is required to:

- prescribe in the best interests of, and appropriately for the patient
- be familiar with the current guidance published in the British National Formulary (BNF)
- be aware of the evidence about clinical effectiveness and cost effectiveness published by NICE
- be familiar with the patient's history, including previous ADRs, medical history, other current medications and any non-prescription medicines
- share information with the patient and clarify any concerns
- ensure that the patient has enough information to make an informed choice about agreeing to the use of the medication
- be satisfied that the patient understands how to take the medication and is able to take it as prescribed
- prescribe the appropriate dosage for the patient
- make arrangements for follow-up.

People with dementia may find it difficult to fully understand or to recall the information they have been given about their medication, so it is important that this information is available in a form that the individual can use and understand. It may be presented in a simple written format, or it may have to be repeated on a regular basis. It is also important for the prescriber to be sure that the person is able to manage their own medication, or that arrangements are in place for any necessary support.

Dispensing

Dispensing medicines is the overall responsibility of a qualified, registered pharmacist. They may work in a community pharmacy or in a hospital.

A pharmacist is responsible for:

- overall checking of a prescription to make sure that it is legal and written by a person qualified to do so
- clinical scrutiny (checking) of a prescription to identify any errors
- dispensing the right quantity of the correct medicine
- ensuring that medicines are correctly labelled with the person's name, the name of the medicine and the dosage
- providing advice and treatment for minor illnesses, injuries and health concerns
- providing a repeat prescription service in cooperation with GP surgeries.

Pharmacists have an important role in making sure that medicines are accurately and correctly dispensed. They are also able to provide information and advice. Most residential homes have a good relationship with a local pharmacist and have arrangements for regular supplies of medicines for residents.

Administration

Giving medicines and helping people to take them is called administration. Ideally, most people should be in control of their own medication and should manage it themselves. However, when people have dementia they may need additional support to be able to do this. The level and type of support that people need may increase over time as their symptoms develop.

Anyone working as a professional in social care must have undertaken training before they can support people to administer medication.

After training they can:

- support people to take tablets, capsules or oral mixtures – oral administration
- apply creams and ointments – topical administration
- insert ear, nose and eye drops
- support people to use inhaled medication.

Additional specialist training is needed before care workers can undertake:

- rectal administration, e.g. suppositories
- injections, e.g. insulin
- **PEG (Percutaneous Endoscopic Gastronomy) feeding**
- giving oxygen.

Key term

PEG (Percutaneous Endoscopic Gastronomy) feeding – a means of giving people nutrition directly into the stomach. It is used when people are unable to swallow.

If you are administering medicines or supporting someone to take their own medicine, you must administer the medicine from the container it was dispensed in. Never put medicines into pots and administer from them, as this can lead to errors and mix-ups. Pills should only be placed into a pot at the point of handing them to someone.

Doing it well

Always make these important checks when you are administering medicine:

- **Right person** – check that the medication you have is for the person you are giving it to.
- **Right medication** – check that this is the medication that is on the person's Medicine Administration Record (MAR).
- **Right dose** – check the dose against the MAR and on the label.
- **Right time** – check that the time is right for the medicine and if there is a requirement for it to be taken before or after food.
- **Right form** – check on the MAR that the medicine is in the form you are expecting – pills, capsules, cream, suspension, etc.
- **Right route** – check that the medicine is being administered through the right route – orally, topically, eye drops, etc.

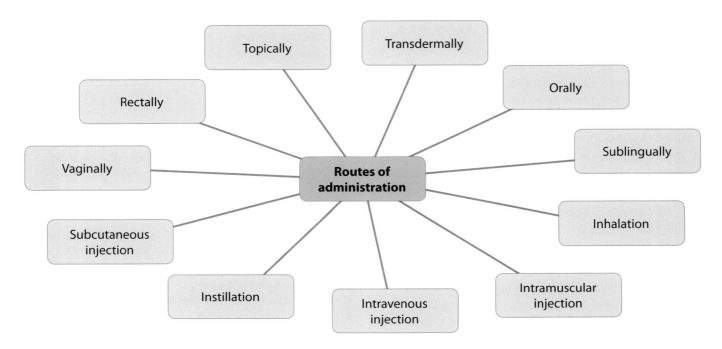

Figure 2.3: Routes of administration

If you are working as a manager or supervisor, you also have responsibilities on behalf of your employer. These responsibilities include ensuring drug safety, record keeping, ensuring that people only administer medications they have been trained for and having clear, accessible policies and procedures for managing and administering medicines.

Consent

Medicine, in general, cannot be given to someone without their consent. Specific steps may be taken to dispense without consent in some circumstances, but this is not the usual approach. Of course, prescribed medication must be offered to the person for whom it has been provided, but they have every right to refuse to take it. Consent, or refusal of consent, should always be a decision that is made with full information. People should know about the medication before they decide to take it, and they should also know about the potential consequences if they refuse it.

If someone persistently refuses to take medication after they have had all the information, the refusal should be recorded and their doctor should be informed.

Some people with dementia may be judged not to have the capacity to make decisions about their medication. In such cases a judgement about capacity will have to be made under the Mental Capacity Act 2005 or the Adults with Incapacity (Scotland) Act 2000. There are five underlying principles about incapacity:

1 A person must be assumed to have capacity unless it is established that he/she lacks it.

2 A person is not to be treated as unable to make a decision unless all practicable steps to help him/her to do so have been have been taken without success.

3 A person is not to be treated as unable to make a decision merely because he/she makes an unwise decision.

4 An act carried out, or a decision made, under this Act for or on behalf of a person who lacks capacity must be carried out, or made, in his/her best interests.

5 Before anything is done or a decision is made, regard must be given to whether its purpose can be as effectively achieved in a way that is less restrictive of the person's rights and freedoms of action.

All ways of supporting people to make decisions must have been tried and found to have failed before a judgement about incapacity can be made. Seeking and gaining consent is important because it confirms people's dignity and rights to make choices about matters that affect their lives. Consent is key to person-centred support.

Being person-centred

The basis of person-centred support is that the person decides how they want their support to be provided and they remain in control. This is as important for people with dementia as for anybody else, and it applies as much to medication as to any other part of people's lives.

Across the UK, all inspectorates and regulators expect support to be provided following standards that include people being in control of their medication. As with all person-centred support, this needs to be built around the needs of the individual concerned and will need to include different levels of support for different people.

For example, some people may be quite happy to administer all their own medication. In this case, if they are in residential provision, their medication needs to be kept in a locked cupboard in their room. Other people may need some level of support, perhaps to open a bottle of pills, but after that they are happy to take their own medicine. Others will need a way of reminding them to take medicines; this could be done using an alarm or a reminder from a support worker. Some people are fine taking some kinds of medication but not others – for example, a person may be able to take tablets, but needs support with their inhaler.

The level and type of support that people need will vary greatly, but it is important to start from the point of the person having maximum control and gradually moving to increase support as it becomes necessary.

Risk assessments

Providing person-centred care does not mean abandoning your duty of care. Working with people who have dementia always means that risks must be weighed against individual choice and control.

Risk assessments will not eliminate risks, but they will identify ways to reduce the risks as much as possible. Care settings must exercise a duty of care and must undertake a risk assessment if someone wants to self-medicate. Good risk assessments do not stop people from doing things; they should enable people to do more because safeguards are put in place to support people in doing what they want. Every person's risk assessment will be different, but some typical areas of risk that could be looked at are shown in Table 2.6.

Table 2.6: Areas covered in a risk assessment

Risk	Approach to reducing the risk
Maintaining a locked medicine cupboard	Safe place for keeping key (key ring attached to handbag or belt)
Remembering when to take medicines	Pager/alarm. Staff reminder
Removing childproof tops	Use plain screw tops
Reading labels	Large print labels
Remembering to take all medicines in the right dose	Use monitored dosage system
Understanding information about medicines	Use reminder cards

Assessment for self-administration

Person's name: ....

DOB: ....

Question	Yes/No	Comment
1. Has self-administration been explained?		
2. Has supply of medication been explained? This should include advice on when to reorder supplies to ensure that medication does not run out.		
3. Does the person understand the requirement for storage of their medicines? E.g. all medicines should be kept locked securely in the drug locker/drawer; the person should keep the key with them.		
4. Has the person been shown their medication with an explanation of the purpose and how it should be taken?		
5. Can the person demonstrate an understanding of: • the name of the preparation • the purpose of the medicine • dose and frequency • when and how often to take PRN medication, and what the maximum dose is?		
6. Has the person been advised to inform staff if they suspect a side effect?		
7. Has the person been advised that they must inform staff if they make a dosage error?		
8. Has the person been advised that they should inform staff of any change in their condition?		
9. Can the person open child-resistant containers, blister packs? If 'no', would the provision of plain caps enable self-administration?		
10. Does the person have good eyesight? If 'no', can this be rectified by the use of spectacles and/or large-print labels?		
11. Does the person have access to a watch or clock?		
12. Is the person able to read and understand written words?		

Special dispensing requirements	✓ if needed	Comment
Tablets out of blisters		
Plain bottle tops		
Large-print labels		
Inhaler aids Is an assessment of inhaler techniques by the asthma nurse/ pharmacist needed? NB. Advise people using corticosteroid inhalers to rinse their mouth out with water after use.		Which?
Individual patient dispensing/MDS		
Reminder cards		

Self-medication approved   Yes/No

Reassessment date: ....

Care staff member's signature	
Name	
Date	
Person's signature	
Date	

Figure 2.4: A self-administration risk assessment form

Case study

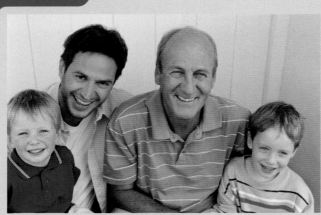

Eric is 76. He has just arrived in a residential care home because his wife died suddenly a few months ago and it then became clear that he was developing Alzheimer's disease. He seems to have got worse since his wife died, but his daughter thinks that her mother was probably covering up much of his confusion. Eric is coping quite well, though he does struggle with words and phrases and sometimes appears with his trousers back to front and a pyjama top instead of a shirt. But he enjoys going to the pub with a few of the other men, he likes pottering in the garden and looks forward to his grandchildren visiting at the weekends – he has their names written on their photos so he doesn't forget them.

Eric has his medication given to him during the medicine rounds each day, when members of staff come into the lounge with a drugs trolley with everything in little pots. They walk round the room and give people their medicines. His daughter asked him what he was taking, but he said he didn't know, he had asked once, but he had forgotten and didn't like to ask again.

1   How would Eric's life be different if he was self-medicating?

2   Has Eric consented to the medications he is taking? If not, why not?

3   What could be done differently to give Eric more person-centred support?

4   What information do you have from the case study that tells you about Eric's capacity to make decisions about his medicine?

All aspects of self-medication need to be considered in the risk assessment. The questions to ask when carrying out a risk assessment are likely to centre around how much information the person has about what is involved, whether they know how to store medicines and all the requirements of locked cupboards. The risk assessment may also look at whether a person can open childproof containers or if plain tops would help, and whether the labels need to be changed so that the person can see them clearly.

If the risk assessment starts from the premise that everyone should be able to self-medicate and seeks to find ways to make it happen rather than to stop it, then it is more likely that the person will be able to maintain a level of control over their life through managing their own medicines.

2.2 Being an advocate

There are different types of **advocacy**.

- Self-advocacy – where someone is supported to speak for themselves.
- Family/friend advocacy – where a relative or friend advocates on someone's behalf.
- Independent advocacy – where a trained advocate works under the relevant incapacity legislation to provide advocacy services that are independent of family or the care provider. These people are known as Independent Mental Capacity Advocates (IMCAs).
- Professional advocacy – where a professional person undertakes the role of advocate. This could be a support worker, social worker, nurse, etc.

Key term

Advocacy – speaking on someone's behalf to help them get what they need.

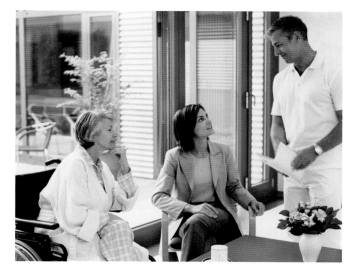

How would you support somebody as their advocate?

Sometimes you may need to undertake the role of professional advocate in order to support people to ask questions or challenge the medication they are being prescribed. Obviously, this is not appropriate if the challenge is to the care provider, but may be helpful if someone wants to challenge the GP or hospital.

There are some issues that are important to understand if you are to advocate on behalf of someone with dementia.

- You must represent the views of the person regardless of whether you agree with them.
- You must not attempt to influence the person or impose your own views.
- People should be empowered to advocate for themselves wherever possible.
- All information is confidential.

It may be important for people with dementia to be able to challenge medicines that have been prescribed, particularly if they are experiencing unwanted side effects or if they are concerned about the consequences of taking the medication. It may also be that someone is unhappy with the form in which their medicine is prescribed. For example, they may not like taking tablets or using an inhaler, and may want to argue for the medicine to be in a different form.

Someone may want to challenge a risk assessment that a care provider has undertaken, for example, a decision that the person should not self-medicate. Clearly, this is not a situation in which it would be right for you to act as an advocate, but you should support the person in organising an independent or a family/friend advocate.

Advocacy regarding ethical issues

You may have to consider providing or arranging advocacy in relation to ethical issues for a range of reasons.

A difficult issue arises when someone decides they no longer wish to continue with treatment, even though this may mean that they will die or their quality of life will become very poor. In this situation, you can only make sure that they have all possible information and have had plenty of opportunity, via an advocate if necessary, to discuss their decision with health professionals, family and friends. Unless there are issues of capacity, the decision is theirs to make.

Another difficult situation is where someone's family requests that medication is stopped because they feel that their relative's quality of life has deteriorated and they should not go on. This is not a decision that families can make on behalf of someone. Many such cases have gone to court for a decision. In the absence of a decision from the person concerned, there can be no question of stopping medicines at the request of their family. There will need to be the involvement of an independent advocate who can act in the best interests of the person.

Other issues can arise over matters of personal or religious convictions. Vegans, vegetarians and some people's religious beliefs mean that they are not willing to take capsules that are made from gelatine, which is an animal-based product. Often this can be resolved by a discussion with the doctor who may be able to prescribe the same medication in a different formulation.

There can be religious and cultural issues around the administration of medications, for example, during fasting. Some medicines need to be taken with food or during the time of fasting when the person cannot take the tablets. These issues can often be resolved, as there are exemptions from the requirements of fasting for people who are ill. It may also be possible to discuss with the doctor the possibility of adjusting the times of the administration.

Advocacy can be very important in promoting person-centred care. Having an advocate makes it possible for someone to exercise choice and control in a situation where they may otherwise have felt powerless.

Overview

Overall, the area of medicines administration is vitally important to people with dementia. It can have a huge influence on their quality of life and the rate of progress of their disease. Getting medication right is vitally important and this can only be done with the consent and involvement of the person concerned. It is your job to ensure that this happens and that people have medication that improves and enhances their lives.

Getting ready for assessment

This is a knowledge chapter, so you will have to demonstrate that you have understood the learning about medication for people with dementia. This unit does not require the demonstration of skills, so does not have to be assessed in the workplace. You may have to prepare an assignment or a presentation, or you could be asked to answer a series of questions, possibly in a professional discussion with your assessor.

Even though this chapter does not assess skills, you should try to relate your learning to the workplace wherever possible. Use examples of people you support (anonymously of course) to illustrate your points, and refer to the medication policies and procedures of your own workplace. Relating the knowledge to your own practice will help to show your assessor that you have understood what you have learned and are going to be able to put it into practice.

Further reading and research

- www.scie.org.uk (Social Care Institute for Excellence: provides knowledge and resources to users of the care services about what works).
- www.npc.nhs.uk (National Prescribing Centre: provides information about the legislation relating to medicines).
- www.mhra.gov.uk/Safetyinformation/Healthcareproviders/Carehomestaff/index.htm (Medicine and Healthcare products Regulatory Agency: a one-stop resource for care home staff).
- www.nice.org.uk (National Institute for Health and Clinical Excellence: publishes guidelines on prescribing medication for people with dementia).
- www.actionforadvcacy.org.uk (information on all types of advocacy, what each does and how to access an advocate).
- www.alzheimersresearchUK.org (Alzheimer's Research UK: the UK's leading dementia research charity).
- www.atdementia.org.uk (AT Dementia: an organisation that provides information on assistive technology that can help people with dementia live more independently. It is particularly useful for information about using equipment to aid medication).
- www.bnf.org (British National Formulary: contains information about all medicines).
- www.dementia.ion.ucl.ac.uk (Dementia Research Centre: one of the UK's leading centres for clinical research into dementia and for trialling new drugs to slow the progression of Alzheimer's disease).
- www.dh.gov.uk/en/Healthcare/Medicinespharmacyandindustry/Prescriptions/TheNon-MedicalPrescribingProgramme (the Department of Health has more information on prescribers who are not doctors, dentists or vets. These can include pharmacists, midwives and nurses).
- www.dh.gov.uk/en/Publichealth/Scientificdevelopmentgeneticsandbioethics/Consent/Consentgeneralinformation/index.htm (further information about consent and key documents relating to consent to treatment forms and guidance).
- www.gmc-uk.org (General Medical Council: more information on the responsibilities of doctors in relation to prescribing medicines).
- www.mims.co.uk (MIMS is a drugs database that contains current information about medicines).
- www.rpharms.com/support-pdfs/handlingmedsocialcare.pdf (this publication from the Royal College of Pharmacists contains further information about administering and handling medication in social care settings in the 'medicines toolkit').

Communication and interactions with people who have dementia

This chapter covers the learning outcomes for both the units. DEM 308 is a knowledge unit and underpins the competence that you will have to demonstrate in the workplace in order to achieve DEM 312.

One of the hardest consequences of having dementia is that people can become very isolated. People may find it difficult to communicate and so stop trying.

There are many ways to communicate with people. Try to see the world from the perspective of the person with dementia, and think about the communication that will suit them best, not you. There are many types of communication; people who struggle to communicate using words will often do so through their behaviour. Behaviour is a means of communication and not a symptom of dementia.

These units underpin everything else you do to support people with dementia. If you are not communicating well, you are not doing your job.

In this unit you will learn about:
- the factors that can influence communication and interactions with individuals who have dementia
- the different ways in which people with dementia may communicate
- the importance of positive interactions
- how to communicate positively with individuals with dementia
- how to use a range of approaches to support positive interactions.

1: Different methods of communicating and factors that affect communication

LO 308:1 312:1 and 2

1.1 Communication through behaviour

308:1.1, 1.2, 312:2.2

People with dementia may struggle to communicate in the same ways as they did before developing the condition. You have learned about non-verbal communication and how important it is in human interactions. In this chapter you will develop your understanding of non-verbal communication further, and learn to understand the possible meaning of some of the behaviours that you will see from people with dementia. Recognising what people's behaviour may mean is like learning a new language. Learning to understand this new language can make a major difference to the life of someone with dementia, when they find that they are understood and their needs are met. It can also make a significant difference to the lives of carers, as people are usually calmer and less troubled if they know that they are understood.

It also helps carers to recognise that people are not being deliberately difficult or awkward. Just accepting this can reduce the levels of frustration that both professional and family carers can feel when behaviours are particularly challenging.

Being restless and unsettled

When a person is restless or unsettled it can indicate that they are unwell or in pain, or it can indicate that they are bored, anxious or angry. Pacing is very common behaviour in people with dementia: it may indicate something as simple as wanting to use the toilet or it could mean that the person is bored and feeling that they need some physical activity. The person may be distressed or angry because they are in a noisy environment after they have been used to living alone; this is quite common when people move into residential or nursing care.

Check if the person needs to use the toilet by guiding them towards it, or if it is exercise that the person is looking for, make sure that they are pacing somewhere that is safe and that they have appropriate clothing if they are outdoors. Well-designed extra care housing and residential facilities designed for people with dementia will have internal 'pathways' where people can pace safely, and many facilities will have safe areas in gardens where people can walk.

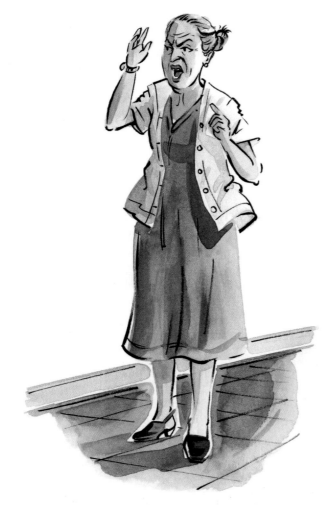

Figure 3.1: How would you deal with this person?

If someone is finding being with others too noisy, try moving them to a quiet area. Sometimes a person may just need reassurance that they are safe – it can be very frightening for someone if the world no longer makes much sense, and a reassuring face, a hug or having a hand to hold can be a huge help.

Many people with dementia will 'fidget': they may pull at their sleeve or constantly smooth their skirt or a handkerchief; some people may repeatedly stroke the arm of a chair or search around in a handbag. Again, this can be a feature of boredom or anxiety. Try giving the person worry beads or a rubber ball to squeeze. A 'treasure box' to rummage in may also be a good way to distract someone from their concerns.

The best response is to consider all the options, then try them out until you find the one that seems to calm the person.

Shouting

People may shout a person's name or may appear very distressed and shout for help. They may wail, howl or scream and they can do this for prolonged periods. Always investigate the possible reasons; it could be that this behaviour is the result of hallucinations caused by medication or changes in the brain due to the particular type of dementia – this will require medical intervention. However, it could be that the person is feeling very lonely, confused and upset. Memory loss may mean that they have forgotten that there are people around and they may feel abandoned or they may be afraid in the dark because they feel alone.

If this distress happens at night, a low nightlight may help and always give reassurance. If someone is shouting for a person from their past, it may help to talk about the person and find out how important they were to the individual.

Repetitive behaviours

People with dementia will often say and do the same things over and over. They may ask the same question repeatedly, for example, asking what the time is, when someone is coming or when you are going out. This is very frustrating for carers, but it is equally frustrating for the person with dementia who feels that they are not being given any information. People may move furniture constantly or pack their bag and then unpack it.

Usually repetitive behaviours are communicating stress and anxiety. Try to give reassurance and comfort to the person. If possible, encourage them to find the answers

to questions themselves, for example, by checking the clock – make sure that there is a clock with figures large and clear enough for the person to read so that you can encourage them to check the time for themselves.

One common repetition is asking to go home; usually this means to a childhood home or a place the person has lived earlier in their life. Clearly this behaviour is telling you that they do not see their present location as home and want to go to somewhere that has all the associations of safety and security. You will need to reassure the person that they are safe and cared for where they are and provide distractions by offering other activities.

Finding out what behaviours are communicating

All behaviour tells us something. It may be telling you that the person:

- is in pain
- is uncomfortable
- needs to go to the toilet
- has experienced brain changes and needs a medical review
- has problems with medication
- is angry and frustrated
- feels lost and scared.

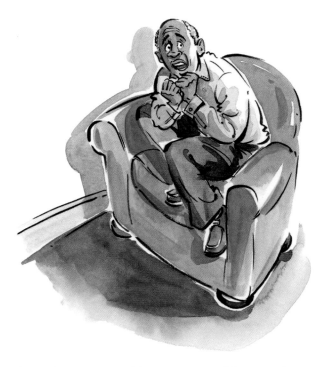

Figure 3.2: How could you reassure this person?

Whatever the behaviour is communicating, you need to take the time to find out what it is and offer the right support to meet the person's needs.

Activity 1

Think about the behaviours identified in this section and add some others from your own experience with people with dementia (for example, uninhibited behaviour in public, hiding things or developing suspicions and frequently challenging or accusing people).

Make a list of behaviours you have seen and then note down the things that a person may be trying to communicate through each type of behaviour.

Reflect

Have you ever been irritated and spoken sharply to someone when they have just asked you the same question for the tenth time in 20 minutes? Have you ever told someone to go away when they have been following you and calling out to you all morning? Have you ever been guilty of thinking that someone is being 'difficult' or 'demanding' because of their behaviour? Would you have done that if instead they had called out, 'I'm frightened and lonely and I don't know where I am. Please help me.'?

Can you see how recognising behaviour as communication will change your practice?

1.2 The importance of communication

308:1.3

Having dementia can make the world confusing and difficult to cope with. Being able to connect with other people is an important way of being reassured that you are not alone and that you are safe and cared for. People may not consciously be looking for reassurance, but everything about their behaviour tells us that this is an important need.

Effective communication is essential in order to understand a person's needs. We need to be sure what a person's immediate and longer-term needs are so that we can offer useful support. It is no use offering reassurance

through hand holding and hugs if someone is shouting because their urinary tract infection has caused them to hallucinate. In the same way, we cannot assume that a medication review is going to work for someone who is crying and wandering at night because they feel lost and abandoned.

Poor-quality and misunderstood communications can lead to real risks for people with dementia: a potentially serious medical condition could go untreated, the person could be left in pain, they may become incontinent, significant changes in their condition may not be picked up or a person could be left feeling bereft and distressed.

For people to have the best possible experience of dementia and to live as well as they can with the condition, we have to make good communication a priority in every support plan. This means understanding a person's individual experience of dementia, as well as trying out all the options when recognising and responding to behaviours as a means of communication.

1.3 Different forms of dementia and communication

308:1.4, 312:1.1

Alzheimer's disease

The short-term memory loss associated with Alzheimer's disease means that people may be unable to remember events that have just happened or they may repeat a question after just a few minutes. Someone may insist that they have to go shopping, even though they have just returned from the shops. This type of memory loss also includes forgetting people – not just having difficulty with names, but forgetting entirely who someone is. This causes significant communication issues, as the person may be unsure who they are talking to, cannot remember earlier parts of a conversation and will repeat parts of a conversation or questions frequently.

Sometimes people may struggle to find the right words to hold a conversation, so they use words that do not sound right in the context. There can often be a link to the word they are trying to remember, but it does make holding a conversation a challenge for them. Struggling to communicate verbally will often result in people trying to communicate through their behaviour; this can often be dismissed as agitation or aggression, thus adding to the frustration that the person with dementia is already experiencing.

Vascular dementia

Although the causes of vascular dementia are different to those of Alzheimer's disease and the brain is affected differently, some of the symptoms are similar, such as memory loss, losing items and disorientation. All of these can create challenges for the person when they try to communicate.

The symptoms of vascular dementia can vary depending on which area of the brain has been affected, but they are likely to include a slower thinking process.

Slower thinking process

Becoming slower in the way that they think will make everything the person does slower and more difficult. It may take quite a while for them to find the right word for a sentence or they may lose track of what they were trying to think of and miss the word completely. This means that communication becomes quite slow and laboured. It can be very frustrating for the person, especially if other people finish their sentences for them – often wrongly.

Dementia with Lewy Bodies (DLB)

Dementia with Lewy Bodies does have some symptoms in common with Alzheimer's disease and vascular dementia, such as memory loss and disorientation, but people with DLB can show some quite distinct symptoms that are not necessarily found in other types of dementia.

Visual hallucinations

Having hallucinations means that people see things that are not really there. The hallucinations are very real to the person seeing them and can cause great distress and fear. It can often be very difficult to comfort and reassure someone who is hallucinating. Any form of hallucination creates major communication difficulties, as the person is not in touch with reality when they are hallucinating. However, hallucinations are real to the person experiencing them so they cannot be dismissed or ignored. Acknowledging the reality of the hallucinations and trying to provide non-verbal comfort and reassurance are the best means of communicating during these episodes. Along with the hallucinations, people can also experience vivid dreams and can move a lot when they are sleeping. Again, it is often hard to offer people comfort after very disturbing dreams.

Differing levels of alertness

People with DLB may show quite different levels of alertness and attention at different times. This can differ from hour to hour and can be very noticeable. Someone who was quite chatty and sharing a cup of coffee and a joke at 11am may not seem to know who you are by early afternoon but be back to discussing the TV programmes in the evening. This means that your communication has to be very flexible and responsive to the person's present state of alertness and concentration. You may have to change from a chatty conversation to reassuring hugs and hand holding in a short space of time.

Fronto-temporal dementia

Fronto-temporal dementia largely affects younger people aged between 30 and 60, although it can sometimes be found in older people. The symptoms are different in many ways from other causes of dementia, although they sometimes look similar in the early stages, especially communication issues such as forgetting words or people's names or not understanding some words. Interestingly, in the early stages, there is no memory loss, although it can seem as if there is because of communication problems. The symptoms can also include personality changes.

Personality changes

People with fronto-temporal dementia may become rude or very impatient. They can also behave quite inappropriately in public, for example, removing clothes or shouting loudly. Quite often there is a change in how someone reacts to other people; they may seem to lose any warmth or concern for others and behave in what seems like a selfish way. These sorts of fundamental personality changes can make communication difficult, especially for those who have known the person before the onset of the dementia; they may feel as if they are trying to interact with a completely different person and struggle to find the points of connection.

2: Positive interactions with people with dementia

LO 308:2, 312:2 and 4

'How you relate to us has a big impact on the course of the disease. You can restore our personhood and give us a sense of being needed and valued. There is a Zulu saying that is very true. "A person is a person through others." Give us reassurance, hugs, support, a meaning in life. Value us for what we can still do and be, and make sure we retain social networks. It is very hard for us to be who we once were, so let us be who we are now and realise the effort we are making to function.'

(Bryden, 2005)

2.1 Ways of communicating to achieve positive interactions

308:2.1, 2.2, 312:2.1, 2.3

Learning about the possible effects of dementia on communication and interactions with others is very important, but you need to remember that everyone has their own experience of dementia. The progress of dementia will have an impact on each individual that will be unique to them. A person's communication will also be affected by factors such as their living environment and their physical condition.

Remember also that dementia is not a single condition; it is a term used to describe the symptoms of a range of conditions. Different conditions cause people to develop different symptoms, but most people with dementia will experience the isolation resulting from increasing difficulties with communication.

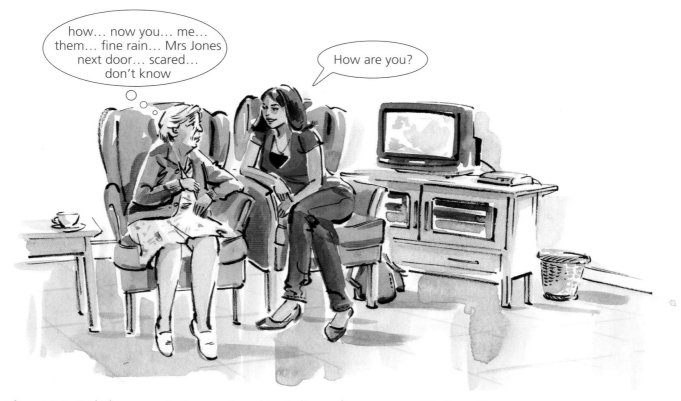

Figure 3.3: Verbal communication can be a big challenge for a person with dementia

Symptoms can cause various difficulties for people with dementia, but the greatest problem is created by people who write off someone with dementia and assume that it is not possible to communicate, or people who give up at the first hurdle and do not bother to try other options if they get no response the first time they try.

Dementia frightens many people; they do not understand it and have ideas that people are 'mad' or dangerous. One man with dementia explained, 'They expect us to be sitting in chairs dribbling and gibbering, and do not understand that we are talking and doing things like everyone else.' Understanding dementia is the first step towards removing fear and to making it more likely that people with dementia are accepted and recognised as being part of communities, neighbourhoods, families and friendship groups.

Of course, the symptoms of dementia do have an impact on how people communicate. They may find it difficult to find the right word for something they want to say or they may repeat something they have already said several times. They may be confused about where they are or what time period they are in. All of these can make communication difficult, but it is certainly not impossible.

Verbal communication

For many people with dementia, finding the right words can be a struggle. Words can be lost completely or may just take time to find. People can also use the wrong word so that a sentence will not make sense. It is easy to feel that there is no point in trying to continue a conversation, but it is important to continue and to make every effort to understand and to make yourself understood. Difficulties with finding words or using wrong words can cause great frustration, especially when the person may not realise that they have used the wrong word and so will repeat it, often getting increasingly irate because the listener does not understand. Often people will speak quite fluently but the content does not make sense to those listening.

When people become disorientated about where they are or about when they are in time, it can have a significant impact on language and spoken communication. Think about how many words you use in ordinary speech that are related to time and place. Some examples are given in Table 3.1.

> **Key term**
>
> **Empathy** – the ability to understand and share the feelings of someone else.

> **Reflect**
>
> Many of the difficulties with communication and interaction with people with dementia arise from the attitudes of those around them. The world of someone with dementia is a different place from what it used to be. It is confusing, sometimes frightening, certainly frustrating and can be very sad. To work well with people with dementia, you need to be able to see the world from their perspective. Do you always do this? Are you sometimes guilty of wanting people to respond to how you see the world?
>
> To help you to reflect on the way you interact with people with dementia, think about this quotation from Tom Kitwood who has been one of the pioneers of person-centred work in this field:
>
> *'As we discover the person who has dementia we also discover something of ourselves. For what we have ultimately to offer is not technical expertise but ordinary faculties raised to a higher level: our power to feel, to give, to stand in the shoes (or sit in the chair) of another.'*
>
> Tom Kitwood (1993: 'Discover the person, not the disease', *Journal of Dementia Care* 1(6), pp. 16–17)
>
> This quotation is talking about **empathy**, which is our ability to recognise and identify with the feelings of another person. If you can do this, you will be able to communicate well with people with dementia. Do not fall into the trap of assuming that because someone cannot express how they are feeling, they do not experience it.
>
> Spend some time thinking about your practice and be honest with yourself about how well you have tried to see the world from the point of view of a person with dementia.

Table 3.1: Examples of words used to talk about time and place.

Place	Time
Here	When
There	Now
Where	Then
Over there	Before
Over here	After
Going	Later
Coming	Soon
Been	This year/week/month
	Next year/week/month
	Today/tomorrow/yesterday

Activity 2

Take a time period of about an hour. See if you can record how many words you say and hear in that period that are related to time and place.

As you think of the words you use, consider how hard it would be to communicate and interact with others if those words meant a different thing to you as to others. When someone is unsure some, or all, of the time about where they are or when it is, it is hard to communicate and interact with others. If people are unsure of where they are, much of what they say may be inappropriate. If they are confused about what stage of their life they are in, they may make comments that make no sense to someone who is clear about the here and now.

When you are communicating verbally with people, you would do well to consider the advice of Christine Boden, an Australian woman with dementia who has written a powerful book called *Who Will I Be When I Die?*. Christine was 49 years old when she was diagnosed with fronto-temporal lobe dementia. This is what she suggests as ways to support communication with people with dementia.

- Give us time to speak. Wait for us to search around that untidy heap on the floor of the brain for the word we want to use. Try not to finish our sentences. Just listen, and don't let us feel embarrassed if we lose the thread of what we say.
- Don't rush us into something because we can't think or speak fast enough to let you know whether we

agree. Try to give us time to respond and to let you know whether we really want to do it.
- When you want to talk to us, think of some way to do this without questions, which can alarm us or make us feel uncomfortable. If we have forgotten something special that happened recently, don't assume it wasn't special for us too. Just give us a gentle prompt – we may just be momentarily blank.
- Don't try too hard to help us remember something that just happened. If it never registered, we are never going to be able to recall it.
- Avoid background noise if you can. If the TV is on, mute it first.
- If children are underfoot, remember we will get tired very easily and find it very hard to concentrate on talking and listening as well. Maybe one child at a time and without background noise would be best.
- Earplugs may be useful if visiting shopping centres or other noisy places.

Written communication

The ability to write can often be lost by people with dementia. To be able to write requires a complex range of skills, including recognising the symbols and letters that make up words, having the motor coordination to transfer them to paper and an ongoing review of what you are writing to ensure that it is communicating what you want to say.

In the same way, reading involves a complex mix of skills, including sufficient eyesight to see what you are reading, the ability to recognise the symbols and letters in front of you and the brain processes to translate what you can see into a communication that you can understand. The reduction in the ability of the brain to process information can often result in people with dementia struggling to make sense of the written word.

This is not true of everyone and for some people with dementia, writing becomes a useful way of expressing themselves. There have been some powerful books and poems written by people with dementia; some of these are included in the further reading at the end of the chapter.

If you are supporting someone who likes to write, you will need to offer them the support that they need to maintain writing as a key way to communicate. If you are writing words to communicate with a person with dementia, make sure that:

- your writing is clear and neat
- it is large enough to be read easily

- you are using a good contrast between the colour of the words and the paper
- you give the person long enough to process the written information.

More than words

Remember that for some people words are not enough and pictures can often be the best way of conducting a positive interaction. The University of Stirling have developed Talking Mats® that help people to use clear and simple symbols to communicate.

Simple cards can also be made quite easily, just as long as people are clear what all the symbols mean and that everyone who is going to use the cards understands how they work. Being prepared to think about the right communication methods is one effective way of showing a commitment to person-centred working.

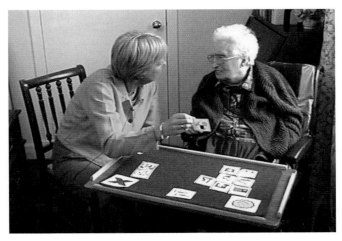

Talking Mats® are used to aid communication.

Non-verbal communication

Non-verbal communication is probably the most important way of communicating and interacting with people with dementia. Only seven per cent of our communication is through words; the remaining 93 per cent is through non-verbal communication.

Professor Tom Kitwood, who was a pioneer of person-centred work with people with dementia, said:

'Dementia sufferers seem sometimes to have a heightened awareness of body language, and often their main meanings may be conveyed nonverbally. In the case of those who are very severely impaired it seems probable that the words and sentences are at times more of an accompaniment or adornment than the vehicle for carrying the significant message.'

Tom Kitwood (1993)

One of the effects of dementia for some people is to make the world a confusing and frightening place. A touch or a kind smile can make a big difference and help to reassure someone who is uncertain. As dementia symptoms progress and people are increasingly affected in different areas of their lives, their ability to communicate is significantly reduced or changed. It is the ability to recognise and respond to these changes that makes good professional care workers, who make a real positive difference to the lives of people with dementia.

As people lose the ability to use language or to process the words they hear from others, then they will communicate more through non-verbal means, so close observation of facial expressions, movements and gestures becomes vital in order to support communication and reduce the sense of isolation experienced by people as their dementia progresses. Non-verbal communication covers many ways of communicating, including:

- facial expression
- eye contact
- tone of voice and the loudness or softness of speech, also how fast or slowly people speak
- touch and physical contact
- body posture and movement
- gestures
- body distance and closeness
- dress, appearance and smell
- use of environment and objects to get a message across
- creative activity, including sculpture, music, painting, dance and movement.

Creative activity has proved to be a useful means of expression for many people, who have found a means to communicate using various art forms.

Positive interactions and well-being

The impact of dementia can close down many aspects of people's lives, but professional social care staff can support people to develop new ways of communicating and maintaining a connection with those around them.

The Bradford Dementia Group, led by Professor Tom Kitwood, developed a set of key aspects of positive interactions that he called 'positive person work'. Positive person work is part of the person-centred approach to dementia care. It is used in a process of 'mapping' dementia care (relating the different aspects of care to a person's life) in order to better understand the world in which each individual lives. Positive person work identifies 'personal enhancers' that support positive interactions, promote the 'personhood' of the person with dementia and improve and enhance their lives. Adopting these personal enhancers will ensure a positive atmosphere in a residential setting and support people with dementia to focus on their strengths and make the most of their abilities. The Bradford Dementia Group also identified a series of 'personal detractors' that reduce the 'personhood' of individuals and reduce the quality of life that people experience in that setting. These 'personal detractors' need to be avoided by those caring for people with dementia.

Personal enhancers and personal detractors are identified using Dementia Care Mapping (DCM). This involves a process of close observation and recording of a group of individuals and their interactions with care staff. The observers have to be trained in how to use the mapping tool and how to provide the feedback to the care staff, but the impact of the way care staff relate to people with dementia and the difference made to their well-being is very significant.

The DCM process usually involves two observers who sit and watch a group of up to five residents for about six hours. Every five minutes they record observations that cover the mood of the residents and the behaviour of the staff. The feedback process can be painful for the staff, but most find it a life-changing experience, as they realise how their behaviour has detracted from people's quality of life. The results can really transform the work of a staff team.

The DCM process can provide valuable feedback for care staff, providing them with essential information about how they can change their practice to make every person's experience more positive.

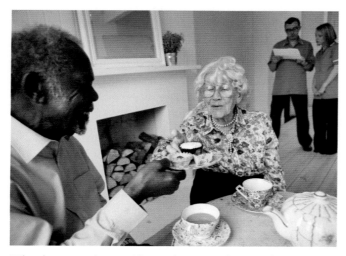

What have you learned from observing the people you support, either formally or informally?

> ### Reflect
>
> A shocking finding in the Alzheimer's society report 'Home from Home' in 2008 was that typically, during a six-hour period of observation, residents spent just two minutes in interactions with staff.
>
> Think about how much time you spend interacting with the people you care for. Is there anything you can change about your practice to help make people feel more valued and cared for?

Details of the DCM approach are given in the Further reading and research section at the end of the chapter so you can explore it in more detail. Undertaking the observations and the feedback can only be done by someone who has been trained in the process, but just looking at some of the enhancers and detractors listed below will help you to think about your own practice and how well your behaviour supports people to live the best life they can with dementia.

The list of enhancers and detractors are from the following source:

Brooker, D. (2006) *Person-centred Dementia Care: Making Services Better*. Jessica Kingsley Publishers, London and Philadelphia.

Personal enhancers – behaviours and attitudes that promote personhood and improve the well-being of people with dementia.

- **Warmth** – showing real care, interest and concern for people.
- **Inclusion** – including people in conversations and activities; not 'talking across' people.
- **Respect** – people are treated with respect as adults and are not labelled.
- **Validation** – people's fears and feelings are acknowledged and taken seriously.
- **Enabling** – people are helped to be active in their own support.
- **Holding** – offering safety and security so that people can be reassured and feel comforted.
- **Celebration** – valuing and recognising people's achievements.
- **Genuineness** – being truthful, clear and honest.
- **Empowerment** – putting people in control of their own lives, letting go of the power of the professional.
- **Belonging** – making sure people feel accepted and part of the community in which they are living.

- **Fun** – enjoying humour and sharing laughter with people, encouraging people to look at the lighter side.
- **Relaxed pace** – taking things at the person's speed, allowing them to set the pace of the activity, whether it is talking, eating or walking.
- **Acceptance** – having positive regard for the person and accepting them for who they are.
- **Acknowledgement** – valuing the unique individual.
- **Facilitation** – providing the right level of support where it is needed.
- **Collaboration** – treating the person as a full and equal partner in whatever activity is going on.

Personal detractors – behaviours and attitudes that take away from personhood and result in 'ill-being' for people with dementia.

- **Intimidation** – making people afraid by using threats or physical power.
- **Withholding** – deliberately avoiding giving attention or comfort.
- **Outpacing** – offering choices or information too quickly for the person to process.
- **Infantilisation** – treating people like children, saying things such as 'there's a good girl' or using a sing-song voice.
- **Labelling** – using a generalisation to refer to someone, saying things like 'he's one of the wanderers'.
- **Disparagement** – telling a person that they are useless or incompetent or stupid.
- **Treachery** – making promises that you have no intention of keeping in order to get a person to do something.

- **Invalidation** – failing to recognise and acknowledge the validity of a person's feelings and perception of reality.
- **Disempowerment** – not allowing to a person to make use of the abilities that they still have.
- **Imposition** – forcing a person to do something they don't want to do or overriding their wishes.
- **Ignoring** – having a conversation as if the person were not there.

Activity 3

Look at each of the behaviours above and make some notes about which of them are part of your practice. Be honest about the negatives as well as the positives. Also think about which of the behaviours you see from your colleagues in your workplace.

Decide what steps you will take to stop the negative behaviours and increase the positive behaviours in your own practice. Think about how you can encourage your colleagues to do the same. You may decide to have a discussion with your line manager.

Doing it well

Getting it right with communication

These guidelines will help you to communicate with the people you care for.
- Show that you are giving your full attention.
- Reduce or stop background noise.
- Speak clearly in a steady, calm way.
- Use short, simple sentences.
- Be prepared to wait for a response.
- Do not finish someone's sentences.
- Listen carefully.
- Observe and respond to body language.
- Be aware of your body language.
- Use touch to reassure and communicate.
- Gently divert conversation away from confused ideas – do not challenge or argue.
- Use pictures or written communication where appropriate.
- Remember to consider someone being in pain or other physical condition that may affect interaction.
- Check glasses, hearing aids and dentures.
- Show genuine respect and care for the person.
- Find out about people's life and history – you will be surprised at how much they have done.

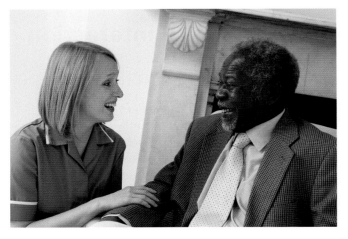

Do you follow the guidelines (right) when communicating with people you support?

2.2 Reality orientation approach versus validation approach

308:2.4, 312:4.1

There are several different approaches to therapeutic work with people with dementia. Two of the best known are reality orientation and validation, which are very different from each other.

Reality orientation

Reality orientation attempts to make sure that people remain in touch with reality for as long as possible. The carers working with the person do as much as they can to make sure that person knows who and where they are, for example, by consistently reminding the person of key facts such as the day and time. This approach uses reminders and notices with calendars and clocks.

People are reminded of the reality if they are confused. For example, if someone keeps talking about having to go home and cook tea for her children, her carer will show her a photograph of her grown-up children and gently remind her that they are now grown-up and she does not need to cook their tea. All activities are done in a way that constantly reminds people of the real world around them.

This approach was very widely used in the recent past, but is not much used today.

Validation

Validation is part of a person-centred approach. In this approach the person's confusion is accepted as being their reality; carers do not correct people or tell them that their feelings are wrong. In this approach the person's emotions (how their experience of reality is making them feel) are recognised and supported. For example, the lady who wants to go home and cook her children's tea will not be reminded of the reality of her situation. Instead, her feelings of anxiety and worry will be recognised; she will be comforted and reassured and then distracted or diverted into another activity.

The validation approach is much more widely used today than the reality orientation approach.

Table 3.2 summarises the main differences between the reality orientation and validation approaches.

Table 3.2: Differences between reality orientation and validation

Reality orientation	Validation
The aim is to re-orientate the person to the present reality.	The aim is to build trust and increase well-being.
Confronts and provides correction for anything that is not based in current reality.	Accepts that there is a valid reality for the individual that may be different from that of the rest of the world.
Both approaches can be used for all people with dementia: individually or in groups or as a way of working in a residential setting.	

3: Factors that influence communication and interaction

LO 308:2 and 3, 312:1, 3 and 4

3.1 Physical and mental health needs

308:3.1, 312:1.2

People who develop dementia do not suddenly become different people. They still have the same background, upbringing and history that they have always had, and they will still have many of the same personality traits that they have always had. Sometimes people with frontal or temporal lobe dementia may undergo a personality change, but for many people, their familiar characteristics will still be there. So someone who has always struggled to communicate and been very shy and lacked confidence is likely to still be reluctant to take the lead in conversations. Someone who was always chatty may still try to reach out and communicate with others, even though their ability to use language in the same way may be less evident.

The work people have done may also be a clue to their style of communication. For example, someone who has had a senior job and was used to giving orders and telling people what to do may still try to do that. Someone who has been a teacher may repeat 'be quiet' or 'sit down' as if talking to class of children. One man with dementia would constantly repeat numbers; it was discovered that he had worked in an abattoir and used to count the animals in.

Physical conditions and pain

People may have conditions such as a hearing or visual impairment that can affect how they communicate. When people have dementia it is easy to forget that communication issues may be due to other factors, and to make the assumption that everything is as a result of the dementia. Hearing or vision problems can be overlooked, so hearing or eye tests may not happen or hearing aid batteries and glasses may not be checked.

A stroke can also result in communication issues similar to those experienced by people with dementia. Following a stroke people can find it difficult to use language and may take time to process communications from others.

Pain

Pain is a major issue for people who have dementia. A study carried out for the Alzheimer's Society found that, following hip replacement surgery, patients with Alzheimer's were given 53 per cent less pain relief than people who did not have dementia. Pain can be difficult for a person with dementia to express or explain. They may not be able to process the pain messages to understand the cause of their discomfort, and so may find it hard to communicate that they are in pain. This needs to be more widely understood by all those working with people with dementia.

Pain can be the result of a range of conditions including:

- arthritis
- constipation
- dental problems or badly fitting dentures
- urinary tract infections
- pressure sores
- tight or uncomfortable clothing

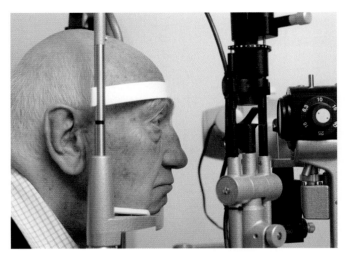

It is important to have regular eye tests to check if glasses need to be changed.

- headaches, for example, caused by wrong prescription glasses
- undiagnosed fractures.

Pain can cause reduced concentration, increased memory loss, increased confusion, aggressive behaviour, sleep disturbance or depression – all of these will have an effect on a person's ability to communicate and to interact with people around them.

Physical disability

Physical disability or illness has to be dealt with according to the nature of the disability. Some conditions, such as cerebral palsy, can also lead to difficulties in speech, although not in comprehension.

Depending on the stage of the dementia, the person may understand perfectly what you are saying but have difficulty in communicating with you. You will have to be prepared to allow additional time for a response, owing to the difficulties that the person may have in producing words, as well as the processing difficulties as a result of the dementia. You may also have to become familiar with the sound of the person's voice and the way in which they communicate. It can be hard to understand people who have illnesses that affect the muscles in their face, throat or larynx. The person may have been provided with assistive technology that will enable them to communicate by producing an electronic 'voice', but technology can become more difficult to operate as dementia progresses.

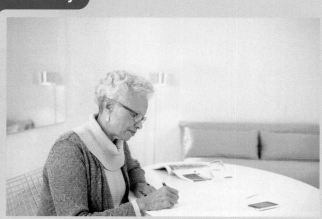

Brenda lives with her daughter Susan. She moved out of her own house as her dementia symptoms meant that she was regularly found wandering in the local town.

Brenda's daughter was becoming increasingly concerned that her mother was able to communicate lass and less; she was finding it harder to get the right words to say what she wanted. Brenda would get her words mixed up and then get very frustrated that she could not be understood. When

Brenda became frustrated, she would scream and bang her fist in the wall.

Susan asked for advice from the dementia adviser, who suggested that using picture cards might help. When Brenda had the cards, she was able to use them to explain what she wanted; seeing the pictures sometimes helped her to remember the word she wanted. Susan gave Brenda some blank cards and she used them to draw some other pictures of different objects. Susan noticed that Brenda seemed much happier when she was drawing and asked her if she would like a sketchbook and some pencils. Brenda said she would. After that she would often draw pictures in her sketchbook and enjoyed showing them to Susan and the rest of the family.

1   How did a person-centred approach help Brenda?

2   What could have happened if Brenda had not been given the cards to help communication?

3   How could you use this example to explain to staff the importance of communication?

Mental health

Depression and anxiety can be symptoms of dementia. Both of these conditions will have an effect on how people are able to respond to others. Depression makes it very hard for people to have an interest in making conversation or to respond to others. Concentration is reduced and poor sleeping patterns can make memory loss and confusion worse. Anxiety can also affect concentration and people can become very distressed as they constantly seek reassurance. This makes any other communication or interaction very difficult.

Learning disability

Where people have a learning disability, you will need to adjust your methods of communicating to take account of the level of disability that they experience. You should have gathered sufficient information about the individual to know the level of understanding that they have. Use this information to help you decide how simply and how often you need to explain things and the sorts of communication that are likely to be the most effective.

Some people with a learning disability respond well to physical contact and are able to relate and communicate

on a physical level more easily than on a verbal level. This will vary between individuals and you must find out the preferred means of communication for the person you are supporting.

3.2 Sensory impairment

308:3.2, 312:1.3

Remember that some people have other communication issues in addition to dementia. For example, some people have hearing loss or a visual impairment.

Hearing loss

Ensure that any means of improving hearing that the person uses, such as a hearing aid, is:

- working properly
- fitted correctly
- installed with fresh, working batteries
- clean
- doing its job properly in terms of improving the person's hearing.

Ensure that you are sitting in a good light, not too far away and that you speak clearly, but do not shout. Shouting simply distorts your face and makes it more difficult for a person with hearing loss to be able to read what you are saying. Some people will lip read, while others will use a form of sign language for understanding. This may be British Sign Language (BSL) or Makaton, which uses signs and symbols. The individual may rely on a combination of lip reading and gestures. Remember, though, that as dementia progresses, people may struggle to communicate using signing or gestures as they did before, as recalling the signs and gestures becomes more difficult.

Visual impairment

One of the most common ways of assisting people who have visual impairment is to provide them with glasses or contact lenses. You need to be sure that these are clean and that they are the correct prescription. You must make sure that people know that they should have

their eyes tested every two years and regularly update their glasses or lenses. A person whose eyesight and requirements for glasses have changed will have difficulty in picking up many of the non-verbal signals that are part of communication. Someone with dementia may well forget about updating their glasses or may even forget to put them on.

If someone has a significant level of visual impairment, announce that you are there by touching them and saying hello, rather than by suddenly beginning to speak. Make sure that you introduce yourself when you come in to a room. It is easy to forget that someone cannot see. A simple 'Hello John, it's Sue' is all that is needed so that you do not shock them.

You may need to use touch more than you would when speaking to a fully sighted person, because they will not see your facial expressions and body language. So, if you are expressing concern or sympathy, it may be appropriate to touch someone's hand or arm, at the same time as saying you are concerned and sympathetic. Having a visual impairment can make the progression of dementia even more frightening and confusing, so being able to maintain communication and interaction is of vital importance.

3.3 Environmental factors

308:3.3, 312:4.3, 4.4

It is important to think past the dementia and look at all the factors that can affect people's communication regardless of whether or not they have dementia. Do not forget everything you have learned about how environmental factors can affect communication. All of this applies as much to people with dementia as anyone else. Noisy rooms can make it hard for people to concentrate, and so can being too hot or too cold. Rooms where others are talking or there is a TV or music playing can make it hard to hear. If someone has the sun in their eyes it can make concentration and communication difficult. All of these are basic considerations that will support improved communication

There is more information in Chapter 5 about how physical environments can support people with dementia and how well-designed buildings and living spaces can make significant improvements to well-being.

Environment is about more than physical buildings and furniture, important as they are. Everything that affects

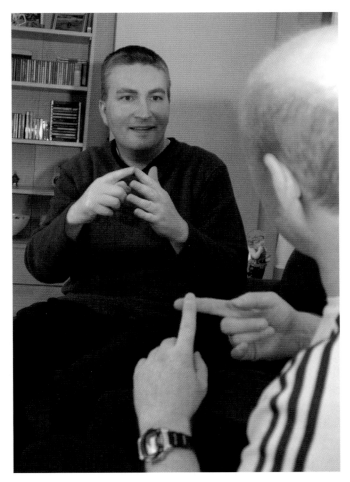

Do you know any words in British Sign Language?

how people live contributes to their environment and has an impact on how well they live with dementia. The following are all aspects of a person's environment that need to be considered:

- staffing levels
- staff attitudes and behaviours
- arrangements for mealtimes
- levels and types of activity
- connections with local community
- level of choice and control for people in a residential setting
- quality and frequency of interactions between support staff and people with dementia.

All of these contribute to the physical and social environment and will have a significant effect on a person's confidence, self-esteem and overall well-being.

3.4 Working with others

308:3.4, 312:1.4

There are likely to be plenty of other people involved with any person with dementia that you are supporting. Some of them will be informal family and friend carers and others will be other professionals who are each supporting the person in some part of their life.

Other professionals could include:

- social worker
- occupational therapist
- speech and language therapist
- pharmacist
- physiotherapist
- nurse
- dementia care adviser
- GP
- psychologist
- psychiatrist
- advocate.

Sometimes it can help interactions to involve another person. This could be because they have a greater knowledge of the person than you do or because they have a particularly good relationship, and the person is more likely to trust them and be relaxed with them.

Alternatively, they may have valuable expertise and information to share. A speech and language

therapist may be able to suggest ways to address some communication issues. A pharmacist or GP may be able to advise on the impact of side effects of medication on how well people can communicate. A social worker may be able to provide useful information about a person's history and family situation that may help to explain particular behaviours or attitudes. The dementia care adviser is likely to be able to direct you to useful guidance to improve interactions and to offer advice. Advocates will be able to offer a view from the perspective if the person with dementia and provide information about the person's capacity and what is considered to be in their best interests.

Of course, not everyone will have all of these professionals involved in supporting them; but it is always valuable to involve them if at all possible so that they can offer help towards positive and useful interactions and relationships.

Family and friends may also be able to support positive contact with someone with dementia. Again, they will have information and advice about the best methods of communication and they may also help the person's confidence.

Always consider if there is something to be gained by involving another person. Any potential sources of assistance in improving and promoting good conversation and relationships are to be welcomed and used to full advantage so that you can be sure that you have done everything possible to put the person with dementia at the centre of your practice.

3.5 Communication and people's unique identity

312:3.2, 4.2, 4.5, 308:2.3

We are all individuals; working in a person-centred way recognises and values each person for what and who they are. One of the problems with traditional approaches to dementia care is that the person's individuality gets forgotten and they are only seen in terms of the damage that is being done by the dementia. All of the aspects of their lives, such as their personality, sense of humour, achievements, kindnesses and family life, disappear as they become a set of symptoms. Person-centred approaches encourage valuing people for who they are and remembering that all the important things about them are still there.

Self-image is about how people see themselves. Would you describe who you are in terms of what you do, for example, a support worker? Or perhaps in terms of your relationships with others, for example, as a wife, a parent or a child? Have you ever described yourself as 'So-and-so's mum', or 'So-and-so's son'? You might think of yourself in terms of your hopes, dreams or ambitions. It is likely that all of these ways of thinking about yourself are part of your self-image.

Key term

Self-image/self-concept – how people see themselves.

Activity 4

Think of four different people who you know well. They can be colleagues or friends or family. Think about the number of different ways you could describe each person. List them all. Do this for each person and see how many of each of the characteristics relates to each of the following areas:

- other people – for example: someone's mum, brother, friend
- what they do – for example: care worker, volunteer at the youth club, gardener
- their values and beliefs – for example: honest, loyal, a Christian, a Muslim
- what they look like – for example: short, brown hair, blue eyes.

Ask each person to do the same for themselves, then compare the results. You may be surprised at the differences between how they see themselves and how you see them.

Identity is about what makes people who they are. Everyone has an image of themselves. It might be a positive image or a negative one overall, but a great many factors contribute to a person's sense of identity. These include:

- gender
- race
- language
- religion
- environment

- family
- friends
- culture
- values and beliefs
- sexuality.

All of these are aspects of our lives that contribute towards our idea of who we are. As a support worker it is essential that you take time to consider how each of the people you work with will have developed their own self-image and identity, and it is important that you recognise and promote this. Just because someone has dementia does not mean that all of this has disappeared and been lost; all of it is just as important as it was before the dementia developed.

Make sure you recognise that the values, beliefs, tastes and preferences which people have are what define them. It is your job to support, nurture and encourage these personal attributes, not ignore and disregard because they are inconvenient, do not fit in with the care system or do not seem to matter because someone has dementia.

Reflect

Think about what opportunities you have in your job to spend time finding out about people's individuality. Be honest about whether you always take the opportunities or whether you find other things to do or decide that other tasks have a greater priority.

Note down some small changes you could make to your practice to make this aspect of your work a greater priority. What impact would this have on the people you support?

Recognising everyone as unique is reinforced by knowing about how they prefer to communicate and what their strengths and skills are. By asking others for information and taking the time to find out about the individual, you are putting the person at the centre of your practice. The information you have gathered will help you to plan the best means of using someone's strengths to support their communication.

Person-centred working

A person-centred approach is all about putting the individual at the centre of everything you do. Instead of making them fit into the system, you adapt and change your practice to meet their needs. This applies as much to communication as to every other aspect of the support you provide. One of the consequences of developing dementia is that people stop being treated as a person; they can lose their 'personhood'. The concept of personhood is about all the essential things that make someone who they are. Professor Tom Kitwood described it as 'A standing or status that is bestowed upon one human being by others in the context of relationship and social being, implying recognition, respect and trust'.

If the focus is on the diseased brain and the losses of memory and function rather than on the positive aspects of the whole person, then that person is devalued and loses their status as a person. Recognising the abilities and strengths that people have rather than what they have lost is the key to supporting them to communicate well and make good relationships with those around them.

Different ways of communicating

Everyone has their own way of communicating. You will communicate differently from your colleagues or your friends or members of your family. Some people are very good at meeting people and talking, others find meeting strangers a nightmare. Some people write letters, articles or reports extremely well and others find it hard to string two sentences together. There are people who are more comfortable giving someone a hug or holding their hand than trying to find the right words.

We are all different in how we communicate and which methods suit us best.

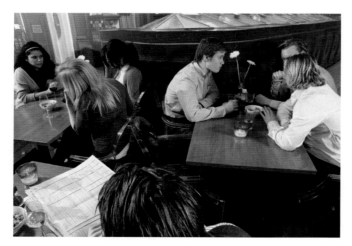

How easy do you find it to talk to strangers?

Everyone has things they are good at and things they are not so good at. Developing dementia will not always change all of that. As different functions are affected as dementia develops, so the skills that people retain will vary, but they are the key to successful communication.

For example, some people may communicate better through touch and facial expressions if they struggle to find the right words. Others may still be able to find words, but may lose track of a conversation, so are good with very short interactions. Some people may have great ability in written communication or even drawing and this can be very useful as a means of communication.

Getting information

Finding out about the strengths that people have is best done by asking and also by observing. Take notice of what people respond to and work out how they like to communicate and what they are good at. Gathering information from other people who are involved is also an essential part of ensuring that you get it right. There are many people you can ask for information – with the permission of the individual, of course. They could include:

- family
- friends
- professional colleagues
- GP
- district nurse
- day centre
- pharmacist
- advocate.

Other people will all have different experiences of interacting with the person, so they should all be able to give you valuable information. Remember to do the following, when asking for information.

- Gain the agreement of the person wherever possible.
- Explain to the person you are asking why you want the information.
- Only ask for the information you need.
- Record any information you are given so that it does not have to be found a second time.

3.6 Memory impairment and the use of verbal language

308:3.5, 312:3.1

Our memories are quite amazing and perform the most complex and challenging processes. Despite all the research that has been carried out in this field, there is still no certainty about how or why memory works as it does. The most widely held view is that there are three important functions of memory:

- **Encoding** – this means receiving and processing information.
- **Storage** – this is about keeping the information permanently somewhere it can be found if needed.
- **Retrieval** – this is the process of recalling information as and when it is needed.

The different types of memory

In order to carry out the complex tasks of encoding, storage and retrieval we all have different types of memory:

- **Sensory memory:** this is a very short memory, literally milliseconds, that we use when we first see or hear something. It is this memory that allows us to look at something and remember how it looks or what it sounds like.
- **Short-term memory:** this contains information that we can remember and recall for short periods of time, usually up to half a minute.
- **Long-term memory:** this is infinite in size and can store and recall information over very long periods of time, sometimes over a whole lifetime. All memories stored for longer than 30 seconds are in the long-term memory.

Long-term memory and short-term memory process and store information in different ways using different parts of the brain: the frontal lobe is involved in short-term memory and the temporal lobe and cerebellum are important for long-term memory. The hippocampus moves information from the short-term to the long-term memory.

Long-term memory

There are different parts to the long-term memory: the key parts are the episodic and semantic memory.

Episodic memory

This holds information about events or 'episodes' in a person's life. Episodic memory holds different types of memories in different ways:

- **Explicit memory** – this is used when we consciously recall events and previous experiences. This means you can remember your holiday, where you were yesterday or an event when you were at school.
- **Implicit memory** – you are not aware of using this part of your memory. It is used to recall information that you use in day-to-day activities without being aware of recalling it. You use implicit memory to do things like brush your teeth, tie a shoelace or drive a car.
- **Procedural memory** – this is used to store information about skills such as making a cake, painting a wall, repairing a car or making a meal.

Semantic memory

The different types of memory are shown in Figure 3.4 on the next page.

Effects of memory loss

As the different parts of the brain are affected during the progress of dementia, so memory function is lost or reduced. Usually, short-term memory is affected most significantly, whereas people are able to recall many areas of their long-term memory.

Unfortunately, it is the short-term memory that is used to deal with experiences in the present. In order to hold a conversation, you have to be able to remember what has just been said so that you can reply. In order to read a sentence in a book or newspaper you need to be able to remember the first part of the sentence you are reading in order to make sense of the ending.

Language is something we all acquire in childhood. There are many different theories about how humans develop language, but broadly it begins at around six months with 'babbling' and continues over the next few years as a learning process until we are fully able to communicate with others.

The reason that we are able to use written or verbal language to communicate is because the information about how to use language is stored in our memories and we are able to recall it in order to use it. The development of dementia can damage the parts of the brain that remember the language we need to use and the right way to use it. It is important to recognise that not all parts of memory will be lost as dementia progresses, and that memory will be lost at different rates. This means that people can be supported to adapt and use the memory functions that they have in order to help communication.

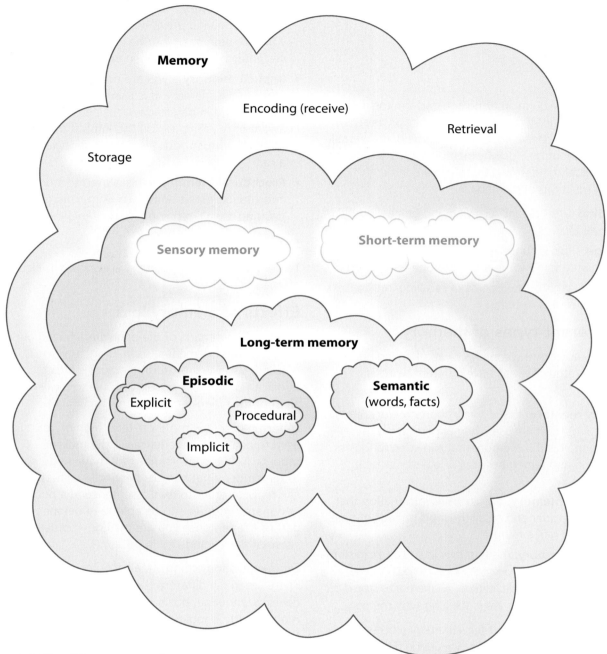

Figure 3.4: The different types of memory

Look at a row of cars in a car park. Then try to recall the order of the colours of as many of them as you can. You are likely to be able to recall between four and seven. This is your short-term memory in action. Try again five minutes later; you will probably recall fewer items than you could originally.

Look at an old family photograph. Try to remember the names of as many people as possible. You will probably recall far more than you could of the objects you have just looked at. This is because it is your long-term memory that is being used to recall the information. Your long-term memory has an infinite storage capacity and can operate recall over a much longer period of time. You will probably recall more names the longer you keep trying to remember, whereas your short-term recall decreased after a short period.

Styles as well as language

We all have a style of communicating that is our usual way of interacting with the world around us. Some people are noisy and chatty, whereas others are quiet and calm. Some people are very tactile and make a lot of physical contact with others, while others are more reserved and use touch very rarely. There are people who are very mobile and active and use many different facial and body movements such as waving their hands around, while others are very still and have very little facial expression. We are all different.

Assuming that you have already done the work to find out people's abilities with communication, you now need to consider how you can best use a person's strengths to make it easier for them to enjoy interaction with you.

For many people with dementia, a spoken conversation is still how they like to communicate. As people progress into the later stages of dementia, they might become less likely to take the initiative and start a conversation, so you may need to be the one who gets the ball rolling.

If you are using verbal communication, you may need to make some changes to your preferred style. For example, if you are usually a person who speaks quickly, you will need to slow down. If you are inclined to ask lots of questions, you need to make sure you ask them one at a time and leave plenty of time for the person to process what you are saying. Use very simple, closed questions which only need a 'yes' or 'no' answer. Avoid long, complicated sentences with interrelated ideas. For example, do not say, 'It's getting near tea time now, isn't it? How about some tea? Have you thought about what you would like?' Instead say, 'Are you hungry? Would you like fish? Would you like chicken?' and so on. Ask just one question at a time and wait for the response, until you have established what meal the person wants.

If you have a loud voice, or tend to shout, think about speaking in a calm way with an even tone. A loud voice or an aggressive sounding tone can cause people to become agitated and distressed. Use very simple, short sentences, speaking slowly and being prepared to wait while the person processes what you have said and composes a reply.

Using touch can be helpful, so if you are someone who tends not to make physical contact, you may need to consciously make the effort to do this. Touch can be reassuring and helps people to get the sense of your meaning, even if they cannot follow every word. In

the same way, body language can convey much of the meaning of what you want to communicate and people can usually read body language very well. If you do not usually think about your body language, then you should try to become more aware of it. Use gestures – they make it easier for people to understand the idea that you are trying to get across.

Many people with dementia have good skills in recognising written words and in using pictures. This can be a valuable way of adapting communication so that people can get the most benefit from using their abilities to interact through visual, rather than spoken, means. Drawing, writing or using flash cards can all help understanding.

Whatever method of communication you use, listening is one of the most important skills that you need to develop. You must be able to listen well regardless of whether you are 'listening' to spoken words, body language, written words or pictures.

Table 3.3 gives some examples of how communication styles can be adapted to support people with dementia.

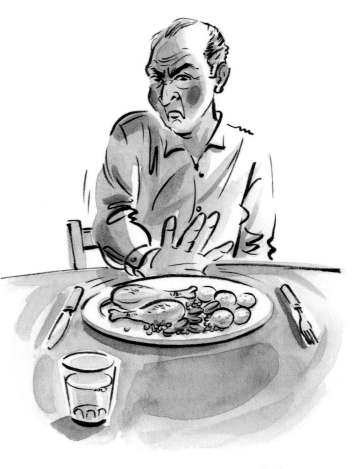

Figure 3.5: How do you think this person feels?

Table 3.3: Examples of adapting communication styles

Style	Adaptation
Loud, quick speech	Slow down your speech and use a calm, even tone.
Complex questions, several questions together	Ask one question with a simple 'yes' or 'no' answer. Leave plenty of time for answers.
Reserved, little touching	Use touch to reassure.
Not much expression or body movement	Use facial expressions, gestures and body movement to help get the message across.
Spoken communication only	Try writing single words, with upper case first letter, then lower case. For example: 'Tea', 'Biscuit', 'Medicine'. Try simple drawings on cards, with a single item on each card.

Communication is the single most important aspect of life for most of us. This is no less so for people with dementia. It is essential that people with dementia are able to reach out and make human contact. This may not be able to happen through language, or any means of communication that most people would recognise, but touches, hugs, smiles, gentle voices and true caring and inclusion will all contribute towards making people with dementia stay in touch with the world around them – even if the world may be a little different to the world that you are in touch with.

Getting ready for assessment

Unit DEM 308 is a knowledge unit. You will be asked to show that you have understood each of the three learning outcomes. This unit does not require the demonstration of skills, so does not have to be assessed in the workplace. You may have to prepare an assignment or a presentation, or you could be asked to answer a series of questions, possibly in a professional discussion with your assessor.

Even though this unit does not assess skills, you should try to relate your learning to the workplace wherever possible: use examples of people you support (anonymously of course) to illustrate your points, and refer to the communication practices of your own workplace wherever possible. Relating the knowledge to your own practice will help to show your assessor that you have understood what you have learned and are going to be able to put it into practice.

Unit DEM 312 is a competence unit and requires you to demonstrate your skills in the workplace. You need to be able to show your assessor that you are able to communicate and interact effectively with people with dementia. Your assessor will also want you to demonstrate that you work in a person-centred way, putting the person at the centre of all your practice. You also need to ensure that you have understood the reasons why you are working in this way and why certain approaches, attitudes and behaviours are likely to result in the best outcomes for people with dementia.

Further reading and research

- www.alzheimers.org.uk (Alzheimer's Society: plenty of information on communicating with people with dementia).
- www.carers.org (Carers Trust: an organisation that supports carers. It provides resources that focus on family carers for people with dementia).
- www.dementiaaction.org.uk (Dementia Action Alliance: an organisation that brings together many organisations committed to working with dementia).
- www.dementiapositive.co.uk (Dementia Positive: the work of John Killick and Kate Allan. It includes useful resources that approach dementia in a positive and constructive way).
- www.scie.org.uk (Social Care Institute for Excellence: click on the Dementia Gateway link to access a large number of resources to support working with people with dementia. There are also useful case studies concerning people with dementia).
- Brooker, D. (2006) *Person-centred Dementia Care: Making Services Better*, Bradford Dementia Group Good Practice Guides, Jessica Kingsley Publishers, London and Philadelphia.

Equality, diversity and inclusion in dementia care practice

This chapter covers the learning outcomes for both units: DEM 310 is a knowledge unit and underpins the competence that you will have to demonstrate in the workplace in order to achieve DEM 313.

It is important to ensure that anyone who uses services is treated equally and fairly and is not discriminated against. Many people find it hard to know how to include people with dementia and so it is easier not to think about them and to ignore them. People do not always understand the needs of a person with dementia and how to make sure that the person is included in all aspects of life.

Anti-discriminatory practice and valuing the differences between people mean learning not to assume that all people with dementia are the same and have the same needs. It involves understanding how to respond to people as individuals and how to put them at the centre of planning and delivery of support.

In this unit you will learn about:

- the concept of diversity and its relevance to working with people with dementia
- the importance of diversity, equality and inclusion in dementia care and support
- how each person's experience of dementia is unique
- how to apply a person-centred approach when supporting people with dementia.

1: The concept of diversity

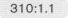
LO 310:1 313:1, 2, 3 and 4

1.1 Meaning of key terms

310:1.1

Diversity

The value of **diversity** is the richness and variety that different people bring to society.

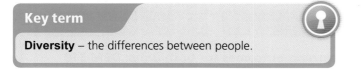

Key term

Diversity – the differences between people.

You only need to walk down the street to see that all people are not the same. There are so many ways in which people differ from each other, for example:

- appearance
- gender
- race
- culture
- ability
- talent
- beliefs.

Imagine how boring life would be if everyone was exactly the same. Science fiction films have explored what it might be like if a whole society was made up of identical 'cloned' people, and this concept seems very unnatural. However, we are not always very good at recognising and valuing the differences in the people we meet.

The work done to develop and promote person-centred working with people with dementia has identified that taking a very detailed life history, and using it in all future planning and work with the person, is central to good practice. Knowing detailed information about a person's past means that you can understand the whole person and see how their personal history has contributed to making them who they are. This 'biography' will also tell you all the special and unique things about them and the individual contributions they have made during their lifetime. This knowledge will help you to recognise and value the diversity among all the people with whom you work.

You can think about diversity in different ways. There are specific differences between people – all of the features that make each of us an individual – and there are broader categories of differences as you can see from the list above. Both of these types of differences are important and you need to take account of each of them. By doing this, you will learn to value the contributions that are made by people's different perspectives, different ways of thinking and different approaches.

Activity 1

Research as many newspapers as you can get hold of for one day, or take the same newspaper every day for a week. See how many articles you can find that take a positive view of diversity, for example, of:

- people who do not match current ideas of being attractive
- people who are immigrants to the UK
- people with a disability
- anyone who is 'different'.

Then look for articles that take a negative view of similar people/groups.

Reflect

When you have done Activity 1, think about how easy or difficult it was to find articles that were positive. Were the positive articles outweighed by the negative? Was there a big difference between newspapers? Why do you think this might be?

Think about how your own views about diversity affect your practice.

Case studies

Akram

Akram is in his late 60s. He is very fit and active and runs a successful small business making car parts. He began to notice that he was becoming forgetful, and his staff became concerned about his concentration and his ability to run the business as well as he had previously done. Akram found that he was struggling to remember the details of orders and that he had forgotten appointments with some of his best customers.

Akram sought medical advice and was diagnosed as being in the early stages of dementia. Once he had begun to come to terms with the diagnosis, he began to tackle it in the same way as he had run his business. He thoroughly researched everything about dementia and created a forward plan. He made some advance decisions and discussed them with his family. He worked out the stage at which he wanted professional caring support and he put financial arrangements in place by making and registering a lasting Power of Attorney for his eldest son. He arranged for his son to take over his business, but decided to remain working as long as he could. He did decide to spend more time on the golf course and less in the office and he and his wife decided to take a long holiday to visit family overseas.

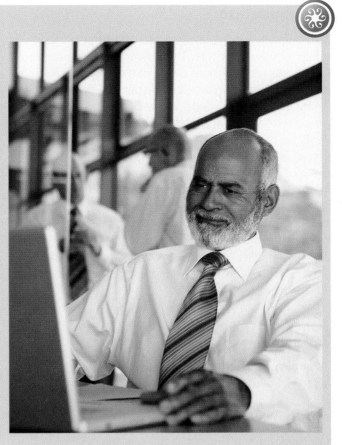

Margaret

Margaret is 83. She was recently diagnosed with Alzheimer's disease after her neighbours became concerned. She had knocked at their door in a dishevelled and very distressed state, saying she was lost and could not find her mother. Margaret lives alone and, as far as the neighbours know, she does not have any family, although one of them thinks that her husband died many years ago. She used to work in the local shop for as long as anyone could remember and only retired about five years ago when it was bought out by a large company and become a mini-supermarket.

The neighbours reported that they had seen increasingly less of Margaret over the past couple of years, but that they hadn't really given it any thought until the day she appeared at their door.

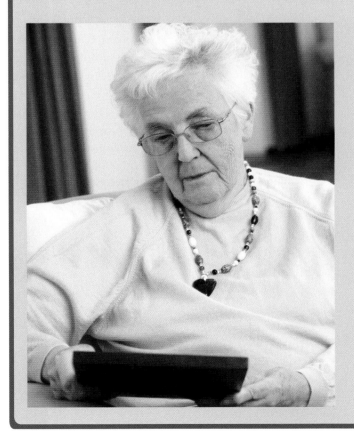

1   Although both Akram and Margaret have dementia, they will need entirely different support. List the care needs of both these people.

2   Explain why the care provision needed by Akram and Margaret will be different. Give examples of why what will work for one of them won't work for the other.

Discrimination

Discrimination is the result of behaviour that excludes, or fails to include, people. This can happen because of thoughtlessness or lack of care, but it is usually the result of thinking in stereotypes. Stereotyping is when we make assumptions that all people in one particular group are the same. Stereotypes are an easy way of thinking about the world. Some examples of stereotypes might be thinking that: all people over 65 are frail and walk with a stick; all young people who live in inner city housing estates are on drugs; all Muslims are terrorists; or all families should have a mother, father and two children. Stereotypes can sometimes be reinforced by the media and by advertising. For example, television programmes might portray violent, criminal characters as young and black, and older people might be presented as dependent and unable to make a useful contribution to society.

Key term

Discrimination – treating a group of people differently from others, usually treating them in a worse way.

If you look back at the case studies on the previous page, you can see that although both of the people have dementia, they are very different, have led very different lives and have completely different needs. If the people responsible for providing their care make the assumption that, because they have dementia, their needs are the same, it is unlikely that either of them will have their needs met.

The effect of stereotypes is to make us jump to conclusions about people. How many times have you felt uneasy seeing a young man with a shaved head walking towards you? Even though you don't know him and know nothing about him, the way he looks might make you form an opinion about him. Try to picture a social worker or a police officer in your mind, then think about how much the media influences the image that you have – do all social workers or all police officers really look like that?

The same applies to the stereotypes about people with dementia. Some common stereotypes about people with dementia are that they sit in chairs mumbling to themselves or wander about getting lost, and that they are completely unable to care for themselves or to have any kind of independence. This stereotype is wrong, in the same way as the stereotype is that all young people wearing hoodies are muggers.

Reflect

Think about the number of generalisations you make every day. How often do you say things like 'They always do …' or 'She never …' or 'Why do people always …' Generalisations are easy to make – and lazy. The danger of assuming that whole groups of people are the same is that you fail to value the differences between people.

Set yourself a goal to reduce the number of generalisations you make, and to identify and think positively about at least one of the differences between people each day.

Anti-discriminatory practice

In order to ensure that the people you support do not suffer discrimination, you need to make sure that you practise in an anti-discriminatory way. Anti-discriminatory practice is what underpins good social care and must form the basis of much of what you do in your day-to-day work with people with dementia. You need to think carefully about how people you support can be subject to discrimination because of the way that they are thought of.

Consider whether activities and day-to-day living in your own workplace are organised without thinking about the individuals involved. Is there an assumption that because everyone has dementia they will all want to do the same things?

Your day-to-day attitudes are important in how effective your anti-discriminatory practice will be, and you need to make sure that you apply the principles across all areas of your work. If you support someone to challenge stereotyping and then return to your own work setting ready to organise all the 'ladies' for a sewing afternoon, you are not using anti-discriminatory practice consistently.

Activity 2

Review your practice, and that of your colleagues, in your workplace over a week. See how many examples of discrimination you can identify. These may be small, unthinking ways in which you or other people discriminate or they could be more serious examples of discrimination. For each example of discrimination you find, think about how anti-discriminatory practice can overcome it.

Effects of discrimination

Discrimination on the grounds of age, gender, race, sexuality or ability can damage a person's **self-esteem** and reduce their ability to develop and maintain a sense of identity. When people are affected by discrimination they experience anger, humiliation, frustration and a feeling of hopelessness. They are made to feel worthless and of less value than others.

> **Key term**
>
> **Self-esteem** – how you value yourself, and therefore how you believe the rest of the world sees you.

Anti-discrimination means positively working to eliminate discrimination and to challenge it if you see it occurring in your place of work. For example, when weekly menus are being planned at a day centre, if no account is taken of the religious and cultural needs of individuals, you should challenge this and suggest changes.

Some obvious types of discriminatory practice are shown in Figure 4.1. You should check your work to make sure that you are not falling into any of these behaviours. You also need to look at the way that colleagues are working and be prepared to challenge discrimination if you see it happening.

You need to develop an interest in learning about other people's lifestyles, cultures and needs. Even though you may hold a different set of values and beliefs from those of the people you support, you have to value them and respect people's rights to hold those values and beliefs. There may, in fact, be occasions when you will have to act as an advocate for someone's beliefs, even if you do not personally agree with them.

> **Reflect**
>
> Stereotypes can influence how you think about someone. Be prepared to challenge your own thinking and assumptions. Don't make judgements about people – try to learn about different cultures, beliefs and lifestyles. Everyone is entitled to their own beliefs and culture. If you do not know about someone's way of life, ask them.
>
> How well do you do this in your own practice? Try to identify the areas where you could improve to make your practice more inclusive.

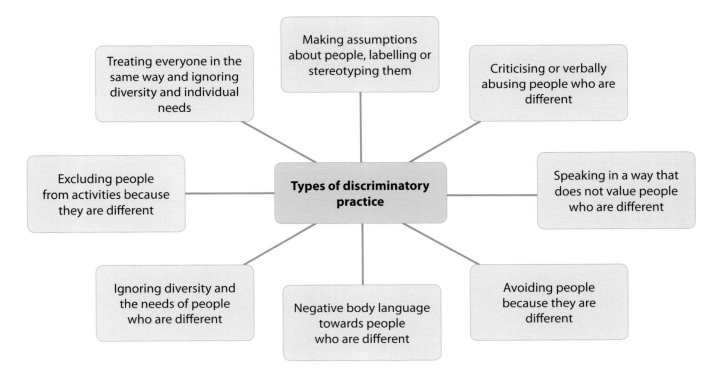

Figure 4.1: Types of discriminatory practice

Oppression

Oppression can be the result of direct and indirect discrimination, but it is mainly the effect of the use and abuse of power on both society as a whole and on individuals.

> **Key term**
>
> **Oppression** – using a position of power to keep people down or to treat them badly.

If you look at the positions of power in the UK such as the boards of directors of large companies, men almost exclusively occupy these posts. According to the Female FTSE Board Report 2010, only 12.5 per cent of the directors of the top 100 companies in the UK are women. The House of Commons currently has 505 male MPs but only 145 women. The average age of an MP is 50, and there are very few disabled MPs. If you look at the characteristics of people in powerful positions, the majority tend to be male, middle aged, white and able bodied.

On the other hand, women make up the majority of workers in low-paid jobs such as retail work, food service and social care, all of which are paid at or around the minimum wage. According to the Equal Pay Unit, women make up 64 per cent of the lowest-paid workers (minimum wage or below) across all jobs, but the percentage is far higher in areas such as food service and social care.

1.2 Heritage

310:1.2, 313:1.1, 3.2, 4.2

Heritage is about more than the genes you inherited from your parents. Of course, this is important, as it influences your appearance, your size, your talents and skills, your pre-disposition to some illnesses and some parts of your personality.

The parts of a person's heritage that interest us here are a person's:

- culture
- history
- personal experiences.

Activity 3

Find out:

- how many disabled MPs there are
- how many women work in social care
- how many women judges there are
- how many women are Chief Constables
- how many people in receipt of benefits are disabled
- how many people in receipt of benefits are aged over 65.

Copy the table and write all the groups of people listed below in the first column, then see if you can fill in the rest of the table.

Group	What power do they have?	What kind of jobs do people in this group usually do/would like to do?	Who can/does oppress them?

- People with dementia
- White, able-bodied men
- People with disabilities
- New immigrants
- People from black minority ethnic (BME) communities
- People with high incomes
- Children and young people
- People who do not speak English as a first language
- Older people
- People with no qualifications
- People with mental health issues
- People who have been in prison
- People who have been to university

See if you can add any more groups to the list and complete the table for them.

This sort of heritage is unique to each person and helps us to find out about what a person with dementia was like before they developed the condition. Any information about the influences on a person's life will help us to see the real person rather than the dementia. The best way of finding out information about a person's heritage is by putting together a life history.

Someone's history is what makes them the person they are now. Just because they have dementia does not mean that they are not still an individual with their own special story about their life, their own likes and dislikes, hopes, fears and dreams, just like everyone else.

Life histories

Putting together a life history is more than just recording a series of the person's life events. These are important, but more needs to be included in order to get a full picture of the individual. The life history should include:

- beliefs and values
- likes and dislikes – not just dietary likes and dislikes but all aspects of life
- important life events, accomplishments, achievements and disappointments
- people who are important – partner, family, friends, neighbours, colleagues
- pets – current and previous
- places and belongings that are important
- the person's skills and talents
- interests and any hobbies – current or previous
- education and work life
- habits and how the person likes to behave
- what makes them happy and what makes them sad
- what they find funny.

The life history should also include anything else that is important in the particular person's life.

Life histories are very useful in helping to make sure that people have their needs met. If you know about a person's background and history, it may help you to understand their present behaviour or to find out about routines that could be useful. It can also help with explaining some of the words or expressions that people may use. Phrases or sayings that the person uses with members of their family may seem odd if you do not know the person. Having the information will help your understanding and improve your ability to communicate well.

If you know about a person's strengths and some of the hardships or great achievements of their lives, it can help you to understand what the person is likely to be able to do for themselves. Understanding a person's history can surprise you – a person who appears frail and vulnerable may actually be very tough and strong emotionally, and may have survived and overcome great hardships.

Overall, taking a life history can help you to see beyond the person's dementia. It will help you get to know someone and to feel more involved with them and their lives.

Life histories can also be useful for younger family members who may have no idea of the life their older relative has led. Looking at a life history can help them to see the real person and understand that there has been much more than the person they see now.

The process of gathering a life history is also a useful one. For many people, the opportunity to talk about their lives is enjoyable and recalling memories and telling you about their past is really beneficial. Do not make the sessions too much like hard work; short sessions over a period of time are better than trying to do it all at once and making someone sit for hours. Depending on the stage of the dementia, sessions of about five minutes may be all that a person can manage, while others may be happy to talk to you for half an hour or more.

There is no set way of gathering and recording a life history. You can use a standard template if your organisation has one. There are some advantages to this, as it means that you know where to look for specific pieces of information. Alternatively, you can use an album style, using a mixture of information, stories, photographs and letters or cards that are important to the person. This can be something that people will enjoy looking through and talking about. For some people, particularly as the generation who use social networking grow older, life histories can be gathered and recorded using mobile technology. Video clips, music and large numbers of photos can be used and easily accessed on devices such as iPads.

A life history can be a good way to share an individual's preferences and interests with other members of staff and other professionals. When it is not practical for others to access the full document, you can still share important information from it at team meetings and reviews.

Case study

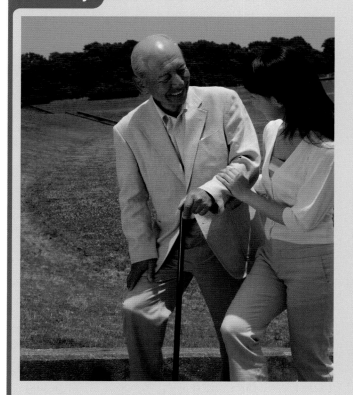

Jack is in the later stages of dementia. He is very disorientated, but is comforted by having his hand held and looking through books on local history with lots of photos. The major difficulty for Jack is that he becomes very agitated and distressed just before breakfast each morning. He begins shouting and trying to get out of the home. Staff always have to spend a fair bit of time to calm him down and get him to come and sit down for breakfast. Staff have tried to work out why breakfast is so upsetting for him and have tried various options, such as serving him in his room and serving him in the lounge, but nothing seems to help him.

In the process of putting together Jack's life history, one of his daughters mentions that he worked in the same office for 50 years and went out to catch the 7.30am train every morning like clockwork. She says that he always left at exactly the same time and was a man who was very orderly and followed strict routines. She says that he was a great dad and did lots of activities with his children, but always as part of a very organised routine. Jack used to have an allotment that he visited on Saturday mornings and also on Thursday evenings in the summer. He would go there regardless of the weather.

The support worker asks his daughter about breakfast and Jack's daughter explains that, in their family, meals were at set times and the menu was the same each week – she says 'That was how Dad liked it'. Breakfast was a family meal like all the others and they all sat down just before 7am and ate breakfast before Dad went out at 7.15 to catch his train.

Knowing Jack's life history has made it much easier to realise the cause of his distress. It is now included in Jack's support plan that every morning someone should go out into the garden with him, just for a short walk. Once he has had his walk, Jack now comes in to eat breakfast quite happily.

1   What are the important messages that came from Jack's life history?
2   What does this tell you about the sort of person Jack is?
3   What needs may this information identify?
4   How does the morning walk help Jack?
5   What might have happened if Jack's life history had not been gathered?

1.3 How people with dementia are subject to discrimination and oppression

310:1.3, 313:2.2, 2.3

Discrimination is caused through prejudice, and prejudice is based on ignorance and fear. People are often afraid of things that are different from what they are used to and that they don't understand. There is a fear of dementia that is based in the fear about mental health. This was reflected in how people with mental health problems used to be treated: they were locked away in institutions, often far away from other people, and people were afraid of them.

When people develop dementia they may begin to behave in ways that are not rational or understandable to many people, and they react by being afraid. Some people will express fear in direct abuse or discriminatory behaviour, but most people will simply refuse to engage with a person with dementia. They avoid people with dementia because they don't know what to say or how to respond.

As a result of being ignored and avoided, people with dementia are not included and can be left out of many activities because discrimination has made it impossible to take part. You can see how people with dementia can be excluded from so much of day-to-day life because they may communicate in a different way from what people expect, or they may not always be clear about where they are in time and place. It is difficult to participate in many of the usual activities if you are not always sure how to make sense of the words you are reading or the numbers on a bus, or if you get confused making choices about what meal you want to eat.

It is probably a combination of our society's attitudes to ageing and a great deal of ignorance and lack of understanding about dementia which contribute to the fear and stigma associated with dementia.

One of the problems caused by the lack of awareness of the true facts about dementia is that people assume that the symptoms are just part of growing old and that there is nothing that can be done. This means that people are reluctant to seek help during the early stages. It is true that dementia cannot be cured, but there is much that can be done to slow the progress and to provide treatments to improve people's health and well-being while they live with dementia. If there were more understanding of the importance of seeking help early, then more people would be able to plan effective ways of living well with dementia.

The government's dementia strategy identifies some key messages that need to be made clear to the general public.

- Dementia is a condition.
- Dementia is common.
- Dementia is not an inevitable consequence of ageing.
- The social environment is important, and quality of life is as much related to the richness of interactions and relationships as it is to the extent of brain disease.
- Dementia is not an immediate death sentence; there is life to be lived with dementia and it can be of good quality.
- There is an immense number of positive things that we can do – as family members, friends and professionals – to improve the quality of life of people with dementia.

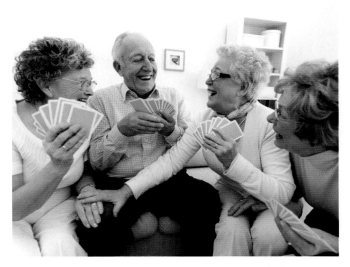

Remember that dementia does not automatically happen to people when they get old.

- People with dementia make, and can continue to make, a positive contribution to their communities.
- Most of us will experience some form of dementia either ourselves or through someone we care about.
- We can all play a part in protecting and supporting people with dementia and their carers.
- Our risk of dementia may be reduced if we protect our general health, for example, by eating a healthy diet, stopping smoking, exercising regularly, drinking less alcohol and generally protecting the brain from injury.

Activity 4

Research work that has been done on attitudes to dementia. You could start with the Alzheimer's Society and the Social Care Institute for Excellence (see the Further reading and research section at the end of this chapter for the websites). When you have looked at some of the research, see if you can think of three different things that you could do in your workplace to change attitudes to dementia:

- among your colleagues
- among the relatives and friends of the people you support
- among the general public in the local community.

The impact of oppression

In order to understand the importance of the effects of placing people in control, you must understand what can happen to people who feel that they are powerless to make choices about their day-to-day activities. How much we value ourselves – our self-esteem – is a result of a combination of factors, but a very important one is the extent of control, or power, we have over our own lives.

Of course, many other factors influence our self-esteem, such as:

- the amount of encouragement and praise we have had from important people in our lives, such as parents, partners and friends
- whether we have positive and happy relationships with other people, such as family and work colleagues
- the amount of stimulation and satisfaction we get from our work – paid or unpaid.

Individuals who are unable to exercise choice and control may very soon suffer lower self-esteem and lose confidence in their own abilities. Unfortunately, they may become convinced that they are unable to do many tasks for themselves, and that they need help in most areas of their day-to-day lives. This can result in people becoming dependent on others and less able to do things for themselves. Once this downward spiral has begun it can be difficult to stop, so it is far better to avoid the things that make it begin.

It is easy to see why people with dementia can feel powerless. As the condition develops and they are increasingly treated as if they have no understanding and are unable to do anything for themselves, or they are ignored and people are embarrassed to interact with them, people's self-esteem starts to disappear and they lose confidence and belief in their own value.

People who have a positive and confident outlook are far more likely to be interested and active in the world around them, while those lacking confidence and belief in their own abilities are more likely to be withdrawn and reluctant to try anything new. It is easy to see how lacking confidence in their own abilities can affect someone's quality of life and reduce their overall health and well-being.

1.4 Challenging discrimination

310:1.4, 313:4.3

It is never easy to be the one who challenges when the rights of people are threatened by discrimination. The problem is that you may be seen as someone who 'can't take a joke' or as 'interfering'. It is not easy to challenge the people with whom you work. However, your professional code of conduct requires you to stand up for the people you support. Most people with dementia are either unable to challenge the behaviour of others themselves or need support to do this. You can do this on a day–to-day basis in your own workplace.

You also need to support your colleagues to work in ways that recognise and respect individuals' beliefs and preferences. Your work setting should be a place in which diversity and difference are acknowledged and respected. You need to set a good example and to make it clear that behaviour such as the following is unacceptable:

- speaking about people in a derogatory way
- speaking to people in a rude or dismissive way
- undermining people's self-esteem and confidence
- patronising and talking down to people
- removing people's right to exercise choice
- failing to recognise and treat people as individuals
- not respecting people's culture, values and beliefs.

If you find that you have colleagues who are regularly practising in a discriminatory way, you need to seek advice from your manager or supervisor.

2: Understand that each individual's experience of dementia is unique

LO 310:2, 313:1 and 3

2.1 Unique needs of people with dementia

310:2.1, 313:3.1

Everyone has unique and individual needs. As you saw in the case studies of Akram and Margaret earlier in this chapter, although two people have the same condition they can have very different needs and make very different choices about how to manage their lives. The purpose of a person-centred approach is to ensure that people are able to make the choices that express their own needs and preferences. A person with dementia is no different from any other person who has support from professional carers, in that they need to be in control of their own lives and the support they receive must be to meet their needs and not the needs of the service.

However, although everyone with dementia is an individual with their own needs, there are some general areas that are common to most people with dementia. One of the big issues that people face is the general lack of understanding about dementia among society as a whole. There is an assumption that people with dementia are incapable of looking after themselves, making any decisions or running their own lives. Nothing could be further from the truth, certainly in the early

stages of dementia, and it is important that there is a greater awareness of what dementia really means and how people can be supported.

People with dementia need local communities to support them. The positive attitudes and involvement of friends, neighbours and local businesses can make a huge difference to whether or not people are able to retain their independence and stay in their own homes. More than with many other conditions, the level of support can make a major difference to how the dementia impacts on people's lives as it progresses.

Examples of how the local community can help people to maintain their independence and make their own choices about their lives include: encouraging neighbours to keep an eye on the person and to know the signs to check for (for example, an open door or milk left on the step); asking the local shop to keep a list of the essential shopping items, so that important items are not forgotten; and asking the local pharmacy to support people with their medication.

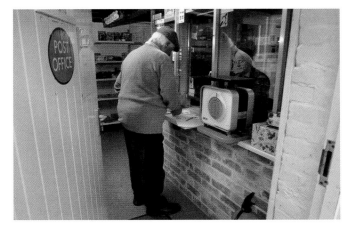

The support of people and businesses in the community is invaluable to those with dementia.

Activity 5

Think of a person you support and make a list of the needs that they have (regardless of whether or not these needs are currently being met). Then add the needs they will have in the foreseeable future.

Make a list of how the person's needs are being or could be met, and how their needs could be met in the future.

2.2 Differences between older and younger people with dementia

310:2.2, 313:1.2

There are many factors that people with dementia share with each other, but there are also a significant number of differences which are based on a range of different circumstances and backgrounds. One of the major differences is the age at which dementia begins. The majority of people with dementia are over the age of 65, but there are considerable numbers of younger people, mainly between the ages of 50 and 65, who have conditions that cause dementia. There are estimated to be around 18,000 younger people with dementia in the UK. This represents about two per cent of all people with dementia, but among people from black and minority ethnic communities who have dementia the figure is about six per cent.

It is difficult to be precise about the ages at which dementia begins, because older people are less likely to have a diagnosis in the early stages, as memory loss and mild confusion are assumed to be part of growing older and are often ignored by people and unrecognised by health professionals. People under the age of 65 who develop symptoms are more likely to seek diagnosis because they do not expect to experience these types of symptoms at their age.

The most frequent form of dementia seen in younger people is frontal lobe dementia, but there are also many people who develop Alzheimer's disease and vascular dementia when they are under the age of 65. Alcohol-related dementia, Korsakoff's syndrome, is more common in younger people, as are Creutzfeldt-Jakob disease (CJD) and HIV-related dementia. For more information on the different forms of dementia, see Chapter 1.

The conditions may be the same as those experienced by older people, but the impact of dementia on younger people can be very different and can result in some quite different needs.

Diagnosis

- It can be difficult to diagnose most forms of dementia in younger people.
- Early onset dementia is not common, so most GPs have little experience in diagnosis. The early stages are often mistaken for depression, the menopause or substance abuse.

- Younger people with dementia do not always fit in with medical specialities, which is where the expertise for dealing with the condition lies, such as mental health and geriatric medicine.
- Early diagnosis is very important, as younger people with dementia are likely to have more commitments and need to be involved in long-term planning as soon as possible.

Personal and family life

- If people with dementia have a dependent family, they need to think about what plans to make for the future.
- Younger people with dementia are more likely to have younger children, who may find it very hard to accept or understand the personality changes that result from dementia.
- Young children lose the support of at least one parent, but often both, as the other parent takes on the role of carer.
- Parents of younger people with dementia may be unwilling to accept the diagnosis, finding it hard to understand how it is possible that it is their child and not them who has dementia.
- Friends and relatives may have difficulty accepting the diagnosis, and there may be less support.
- Changes in sexual interest – either a reduction or loss of interest or increased sexual demands – may cause relationship problems.
- Personality changes can cause challenges for families.

Behaviour

- Younger people with dementia may still be more active and energetic, so the changes in behaviour, such as wandering or aggressive outbursts, can be more challenging.
- Younger people with dementia are often unwilling to give up driving, as this reduces their independence. However, people with dementia should not drive and are unlikely to be able to get insurance following diagnosis.
- There is a lack of awareness among the public of early onset dementia, so behaviours may not be tolerated in the same way as they would with an older person.
- Behaviours can lead to issues such as being arrested for shoplifting, which is less likely to be recognised as a symptom of dementia than it would be with an older person.

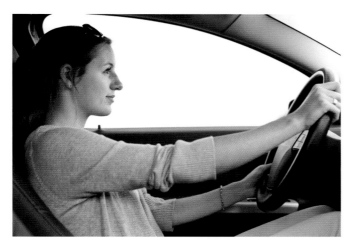

Do you drive? How would you feel if your licence and car were taken away from you?

Employment

- It is more likely that the person will be unable to continue working.

- The person is unlikely to be receiving a state or occupational pension, so they need to ensure they claim all benefits due to them.

- The person's partner may also have to leave work to become the person's carer, resulting in serious loss of income and changes in lifestyle.

Legal and financial matters

- Younger people are more likely to have a living partner, therefore issues such as joint bank accounts need to be dealt with.

- People are more likely to have financial commitments such as mortgages.

- Plans need to be made to consider lasting power of attorney in relation to health and welfare or property and financial affairs. The arrangements are similar, but slightly different, for people living in Scotland.

2.3 The effect of an individual's experience of dementia on carers

310:2.3, 313:1.4

Many carers have been undertaking their caring role for a long time and are well used to meeting the needs of their loved one. However, sometimes the very closeness can mean that needs are not always recognised or preferences acted upon. You will often hear 'We always do it like this', 'He prefers it this way' or 'She doesn't like to …' This is not because people are unthinking, but because caring for someone with dementia is very demanding, and continuing to do things as they have always been done may seem the easier way rather than risk trying anything new.

Working closely with carers so that they are able to recognise the value of person-centred working is important and rewarding. Often carers will be amazed and delighted at the change in the person they love as they learn how to meet individual needs by responding to behaviour as a means of communication rather than seeing it a symptom of the dementia.

Being a carer can be a very lonely life. When carers are introduced to the idea of support being provided by the local community, it can take a huge load from their shoulders and they may welcome involvement from others. Carers often believe that caring for their loved one is something they must do themselves and are reluctant to ask for help. Finding that there are other people willing to offer support can be a great relief.

It is not always easy for people to reach the view that there may be another way of doing things, especially if they have been caring for a long time. The best way is always to show people person-centred approaches in action, perhaps by arranging a visit to a local facility which uses a person-centred approach. It is always easier to show people

Activity 6

Research how many younger people (people under the age of 65) with dementia there are in your local area. It may not be easy to find out and you may have to ask both your local primary care trust (PCT) and the local authority's Adult Services department. If you have a local branch of the Alzheimer's Society, they may have the information.

- Once you know the approximate numbers, find out what services are available for younger people with

dementia in your area. You will need to find out what is offered by local GPs, hospitals and social services. Check if there are any local voluntary organisations or support groups for people with dementia and their carers. Find out how younger people can access the services and how many people use them. How difficult was it to find services?

- How do you think services could be improved?

something in practice rather than just trying to explain. It is also important to take the time to explain how this approach will work with their own loved one. If you are supporting the person, you can demonstrate through your own actions the difference it can make when a person's unique needs are recognised and responded to.

Everyone likes information in a way that suits them. Some people will welcome written information about the way you are working, while others will want a verbal discussion and the opportunity to look through written information later. If you have the task of explaining person-centred approaches to a carer, make sure that you find out the best way to give them the information. Use your communication skills to give information in a way that does not appear to criticise how they are currently caring for their loved one with dementia and be sensitive to how some people may respond if they feel that they are not being valued and appreciated.

Above all, you need to make sure that carers can see the possible benefits for all concerned of putting the person with dementia in control of their life and in control of making sure that their needs are known and that everyone understands their preferences about how to meet them.

Doing it well

Communicating with carers
- Be sensitive to people's feelings.
- Value the work they are doing.
- Explain and give information in a way that people can use.
- Back up verbal information with written details.
- Show people how the approach works in action if they wish.
- Use your own work as an example.

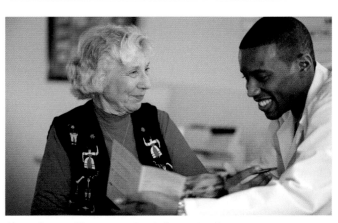

How do you like to receive information?

2.4 How the experience of dementia may be different for individuals

310:2.4, 313:1.3

Learning disabilities and dementia

As a result of advances in medical and social care, people with learning disabilities are living longer and are in better health than previously. Therefore, more people with a learning disability are living into older age and developing the conditions associated with ageing, including dementia.

There is a known connection between Down's syndrome and dementia. People with Down's have a much higher chance of developing dementia at a younger age than the rest of the population and than people with different types of learning disability. The risk is three or four times higher than for the general population. The most common form of dementia experienced by people with Down's syndrome is Alzheimer's disease.

Studies have shown that the numbers of people with Down's syndrome who have Alzheimer's disease are approximately:

- 1 in 50 of those aged 30 to 39 years
- 1 in 10 of those aged 40 to 49 years
- 1 in 3 of those aged 50 to 59 years
- more than half of those who live to 60 or over.

The reasons for this are not completely understood as yet, but it seems likely that the proteins that change the brain in Alzheimer's disease have a genetic link to the chromosome that causes Down's syndrome.

Studies suggest that the numbers of people with learning disabilities other than Down's syndrome who have dementia are approximately:

- 1 in 10 of those aged 50 to 65
- 1 in 7 of those aged 65 to 75
- 1 in 4 of those aged 75 to 85
- nearly three-quarters of those aged 85 or over.

The figures show that there is a very high incidence of younger people with a learning disability who develop dementia in comparison to the general population. Many of them will experience the same sorts of issues as younger people without a learning disability (see pages 74–75), but there are some differences:

- There are some different signs and symptoms in the early stages. For example, among people with Down's syndrome, changes in behaviour are more likely to be noticed initially than memory loss. People are reported as becoming withdrawn or very stubborn and irritable. Epilepsy is more common among people with Down's syndrome than in the general population, but if a person only begins to have fits in later life, it is often a symptom of dementia.

- People with a learning disability are less likely to receive an early diagnosis of dementia. Health professionals or carers may not recognise the start of dementia, although there is widespread awareness of the link between Alzheimer's and Down's.

- People with Down's syndrome may have difficulty in understanding the implications of a diagnosis of dementia and can find the changes in their own behaviour and abilities confusing and frustrating. The person and/or their family are likely to require specific support to understand the changes, and to make sure they can access appropriate services after diagnosis and as dementia progresses.

- There may be a more rapid progression of dementia. The stages of dementia are the same for people with Down's as for the general population, but the move into each stage may be quicker.

- The person may already be in a supported living environment, or be supported by family. The changes as dementia develops may make it a challenge for the person to remain in their usual living environment as additional support may be needed.

- The person may already have a communication plan in place, depending on the severity and nature of the learning disability.

- The person may already have support in place and regular contact with social work, community, day, residential or housing services.

Diagnosing dementia

Diagnosis will vary depending on the severity of the learning disability. Because diagnosis of dementia is based on changes in behaviour rather than increasing memory loss and confusion, it is important to take very detailed information from families or support workers to identify how and when changes began to happen. There will also have to be a full health assessment to rule out any physical causes. People with a learning disability have an annual health check with their GP, so this is a good opportunity to examine any changes in behaviour that may indicate the start of dementia.

Working in a person-centred way

The principles of person-centred working apply in the same way when working with people with a learning disability. In fact, person-centred working was pioneered in the learning disability sector, so people should be used to making support plans and being in control of their own lives and support.

Many people with a learning disability will already have a life history and a personal profile. A diagnosis of dementia will mean that support plans should be reviewed so that the implications of the dementia diagnosis can be included. All of the important areas of person-centred work with people with dementia, such as history, local community and physical abilities, are just as important and need to be looked at as part of a revised plan.

In the early stages, people will still be able to continue with most of the activities they have enjoyed; sport, walking, art, gardening and so on should be encouraged. During the later stages, the range of activities may be reduced and new ones introduced. Careful future planning can help to make smooth transitions as people progress through the stages of dementia, especially as this can be a quicker progression than for people without a learning disability.

Activity 7

This is a similar activity to Activity 6, in which you found out about the number of younger people with dementia in your local area. Now find out the number of people with a learning disability who have dementia. This should be easier, as most people with a learning disability have services from the local authority's Adult Services.

When you know the numbers, find out what services are available for people with a learning disability who have dementia. You will need to find out what is offered by local GPs, hospitals and social services. Check if there are any local voluntary organisations or support groups for people with a learning disability with dementia and their carers. Find out how people can access the services and how many people use them.

- How difficult was it to find services?
- How do you think services could be improved?

Dementia among people of different ethnic backgrounds

Everyone's experience of dementia is different and unique to them, but there are certain factors that influence the experience of different people. A person's ethnic and cultural background is one of these factors. Working with people from a black and minority ethnic (BME) community means that you need to understand how dementia is viewed within that community and the likely impact on the way the condition is managed and supported.

The latest estimates in the government's dementia strategy, *Living Well with Dementia* (2009), are that there are about 15,000 people from BME communities currently with dementia. This is expected to rise considerably in the next few years, as people who arrived in the UK during the 1950s, 1960s and 1970s are reaching older age. There is little hard evidence about the frequency of dementia in various BME populations, but it is thought that vascular dementia is more common among Asian and black Caribbean groups because they are more likely to have the diseases that cause higher risks of dementia, such as cardiovascular disease, diabetes and high blood pressure.

How dementia is viewed

There seems to be evidence that awareness of dementia is low among black Caribbean communities and, interestingly, there is no word for dementia in many South Asian languages. There is a tendency among BME communities to consider that the symptoms of dementia are part of normal ageing and to assume that nothing can be done. This can often mean that people only ask for help when dementia is quite advanced, reducing people's opportunity to make choices and decisions about their support.

There is a stigma attached to dementia in all cultures, but this can be more obvious in some BME communities. For example, in some Asian religious groups dementia may be viewed as a punishment for past lives and in black Caribbean communities it is more likely to be viewed as a mental illness rather than as changes to the brain. In communities where there are arranged marriages, having a family member with dementia might affect the marriage prospects of younger family members. There is some evidence that in Eastern European communities the stigma of dementia is linked to previous experiences of persecution.

A study that compared the elements of life that were important to people with dementia found that white British people with dementia were most concerned about retaining independence for as long as possible, black Caribbean people were concerned about being a burden to their families and Asian people valued family support and were proud of it.

Life histories

Life histories are very important when working with people from BME communities because they will help you to make sure that you are responding to the person as an individual and not using racial or ethnic stereotypes to assess their needs. Many of the people who are developing dementia now were not born in the UK. This makes recording their life history even more important, because there will be important parts of their lives that took place in another country and the process of migration will be a key memory. In the future, there will be far more people from BME communities who were born in the UK, so their life histories will not have this element.

Carers

Some research that has been carried out among carers in BME communities has shown that there is a very high expectation that women and adult children will undertake caring. It has been found that people in some BME communities do not see themselves as 'carers' as such. The concept of caring for a family member is just part of the obligations and duty of kinship. This is one reason why people may be reluctant to seek support. They may also be concerned that services will not meet the same standards as family care or that they will be criticised within the community for using services rather than providing family support.

However, increasingly, women from BME communities are also working and so it is more difficult for them to undertake the traditional caring roles.

Working with people from different ethnic backgrounds

The basic requirements of working well with people from backgrounds and cultures that are different to your own are the same, regardless of the user group. You need to ensure that you find out information about the cultural and religious needs of the individual and you need to familiarise yourself with basic words in the person's language. Do not forget that people who speak English as a second language may lose the ability to speak it as their dementia progresses. Ensure that communication is undertaken in the language that the person can use and understand.

It is important that social activities are appropriate and that all cultural dietary needs are considered. Consultation with the person, their family and their local community is important to be sure that you are providing a service that will meet the person's needs.

Activity 8

Research how many people from BME communities use dementia services in your local area. It may not be easy to find out and you may have to ask both your PCT and your local authority's Adult Services. You will also need to see if you can find out this information from local voluntary organisations who work in BME communities. If your local area does not have a significant BME population, then research another one that does.

Once you know the approximate numbers, find out what services are available in your area for people from BME communities. This means services specifically aimed at people from particular communities, not mainstream services that happen to be used by people from a particular BME community. This will vary depending on where you live. Try voluntary groups, social services and health services. Include residential services, day care services, domiciliary care services, specialist housing, advocacy, rights advice and befriending services.

● How difficult was it to find services?
● How do you think services could be improved?

End-of-life care

The National Council for Palliative Care defines end-of-life care as care that:

'helps all those with advanced, progressive, incurable illness to live as well as possible until they die. It enables the supportive and palliative care needs of both patient and family to be identified and met throughout the last phase of life and into bereavement. It includes management of pain and other symptoms and provision of psychological, social, spiritual and practical support.'

(Source: National Council for Palliative Care, 2006)

Of the half a million people who die each year, 58 per cent die in hospital, 18 per cent at home, 17 per cent in care homes, 4 per cent in hospices and 3 per cent elsewhere. How, when and where we die has changed significantly in the UK over the past 100 years. In 1900 most people died at home and many died far younger than today, when 66 per cent of people who die are aged over 75.

Providing high-quality care at the end of a person's life is important. For many people with life-limiting illnesses such as cancer, it is possible to plan and to work alongside the person so that they have the death that they want. For many people with dementia it is more complex. It may not be possible to find out what people want, they may not understand what is happening to them and it can be difficult to be sure when symptoms change to indicate that the end of life is approaching.

Advance decisions are very useful at the end of a person's life. If they have already shared their wishes with their family or with those providing support, it is easier to be sure that you are doing what the person wanted. The Department of Health has developed an End of Life Care Pathway (see Figure 4.2) that identifies the key steps to supporting a person at the end of their life:

Steps 1 and 2 can present difficulties for people with dementia if there have not been any advance decisions. Family and friends can sometimes provide information about people's wishes and advocates can support communication if necessary. Remember to use the information you have gathered from a person's life history to think about their values and cultural needs at the end of their life.

People should be kept free from pain and as comfortable as possible during the end of life. They should also be given comfort and human contact. If family and loved ones are there, they will do this and should be encouraged to talk to the person and make contact by holding their hands and stroking. If there is no family there, then support staff should ensure that people do not die alone and unsupported.

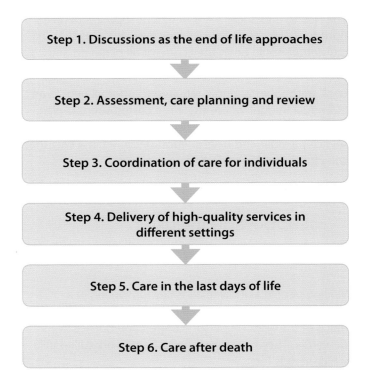

Figure 4.2: Care Pathway

3: Understand the importance of working in a person-centred way and how this links to inclusion

LO 310:3, 313:2, 3 and 4

3.1 Legislation

310:3.1, 313:2.1

The Equality Act 2010 replaces all the previous pieces of legislation regarding equality, such as the Race Relations Act, the Sex Discrimination Act and the Equal Pay Act. It extends those protected by the Act to include older people. The Act also gives protection to people not to be discriminated against on the grounds of their sexual orientation.

The broad aim of the Equality Act is to protect the rights of individuals and to provide equality of opportunity. For more information on the Equality Act, see Chapter 5, pages 89–90.

Human rights are protected by the Human Rights Act 1998, which is covered in detail in Chapter 5 on pages 86–89.

The Health and Social Care Act 2012 supports people's right to make choices about their lives. It states that the individual should be at the centre of all planning and delivery of services.

Local authorities are now required to offer all people an Individual Budget where there is a costed support plan, and people are given the funding to choose their own service provider and have support delivered in a way that suits them and the way they want to live.

3.2 Meeting individual needs and supporting inclusion

310:3.2, 3.3, 3.4, 313:2.4, 3.3, 3.4, 4.1

Valuing people as individuals is key to working in a person-centred way. Bradford University has developed much of the work on person-centred approaches to dementia. They have developed a framework called VIPS, which stands for:

- **Valuing** – unconditional valuing of the person with dementia, their carers and the professional staff. This means valuing everyone and recognising that person-centred approaches are about everyone involved – not just the person with dementia.
- **Individualised** – recognising and responding to the person as a unique individual.
- **Perspective** – seeing the world from the person's view point.
- **Supportive** – making sure that the person's environment is positive and supports their well-being.

Factors that inhibit inclusion

It is easy to forget the factors that can make people with dementia feel that they do not belong, or that they cannot participate in what is going on around them. These factors can be simple things, such as:

- people talking too quickly before the person can process the information
- asking too many questions
- information in a format or style that the person cannot understand
- a situation with lots of people the person does not know
- being in a strange place.

Other factors can be more complex and harder to resolve, such as:

- a complicated system to access services
- buildings with a confusing design
- unsupportive local community
- a local area that is not easy to walk around in
- service providers that keep changing staff.

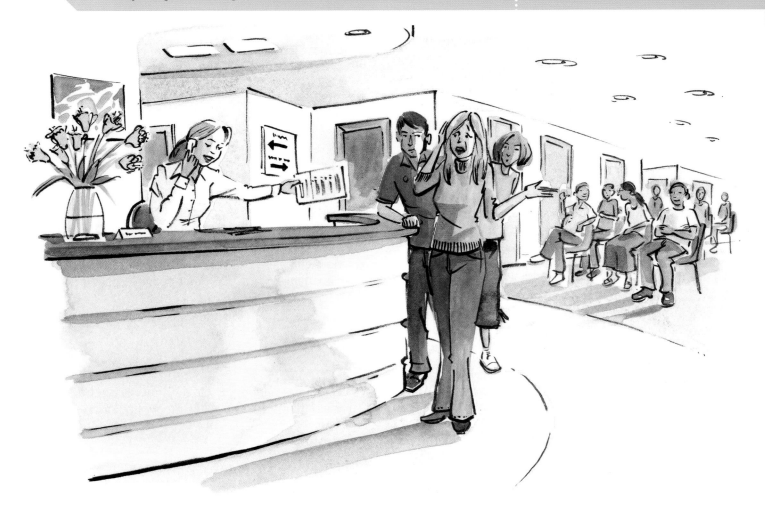

Figure 4.3: How do you think a person with dementia might feel in this environment?

Although it may be easier to sort out the simpler things, the more difficult issues do need to be addressed if people are to be able to feel that they are included and involved. You may not be able to solve issues personally, but you do have a responsibility to report issues that are causing people to feel excluded and to highlight them to your line managers so that problems can be considered. There is a strong chance that organisations that fail to value people or that fail to work in an inclusive way will result in discrimination against individuals or against a whole group of people.

Supporting people to make their own choices

Social care has moved on from the days when we did things 'to' people and provided people with whatever we, as professionals, considered to be best for them. Over the last few years, we have come to understand

that needing support from social care professionals does not mean that you have to give up choice and control over your life.

It is important that people are involved in all aspects of their lives and not just passive receivers of 'care'. Involving people is not just about deciding on support packages, but is also about making sure that people have a real input into what happens to them on a day-to-day basis, from choosing clothes to self-medication. It is also about issues such as deciding when and where to go out, when to get up and when to go to bed, and how to spend free time.

An individual's ability to be involved in all the different aspects of their support will vary depending on the stage and nature of their dementia and some people's ability to participate may fluctuate. However, the opportunity should always be there and nothing should be done without offering the person the chance to state their views. Someone in the early stages of dementia may be able to state their wishes very clearly and be able to enter into discussions around some of the bigger issues. A person in the later stages may find that difficult, but may still be able to understand and communicate using various techniques, including responding to simple questions or using flash cards, pictures and touch.

Working in this way when people have dementia does have risks, and these must be taken into account. For example, everyone should be encouraged to self-medicate, but all the risks have to be taken into account. Someone in the early stages of dementia can be supported to manage their own medication for as long as possible, whereas someone who is in the later stages of dementia and who is very disorientated with serious memory loss would not be able to be responsible for their own medication. However, they should still have the opportunity to be involved as far as possible, even if it is simply by physically taking their own medication rather than having it put in their mouth by someone else.

As you work with someone with dementia, you will become quite skilled at communicating with them, so it will be possible for you to seek their views and wishes about day-to-day aspects of their life. Questions will need to be straightforward and only require a simple answer, but the information that you know about the person from their life history will help.

For example, if you know someone has been a keen gardener and you are asking about how they would like to spend the afternoon, you could try asking, 'Would you like to come and sit in the garden?' For someone in the later stages of dementia do not ask, 'What would you like to do this afternoon?' The question is too complex and hard for the person to process.

The support that people have selected in order to help them to live well with their dementia is not only about day–to-day living and personal care. There are also bigger issues, such as how people relate to their local community, which family members and friends they want to see regularly and how they want to socialise with others. There are also important discussions around medicines, treatment and how people wish to experience the end of their life. These elements of support should be discussed and the person's wishes recorded as early as possible in the course of their dementia so that you can be sure that you are able to find out their wishes.

Supporting inclusion

Inclusion involves making sure that people are included and not left out. Supporting people to take part in society is supporting inclusion. Often, ensuring that people are included is about moving barriers that are in the way and stopping people from taking part. There can be many different sorts of barriers to inclusion:

- physical barriers, such as problems with access
- intellectual barriers: people may be excluded because they cannot respond or participate quickly as a result of conditions such as dementia
- language barriers: either speaking a different language or using jargon that people cannot understand
- financial barriers: costs can mean that some people cannot take part
- emotional barriers: people may feel intimidated or lack confidence
- lack of information: people may not realise that certain things are available or know how to access them.

Inclusive practice is about ensuring that there are no barriers that would exclude people or make it difficult for them to participate fully in society. People must be included in all aspects of life, not excluded from some of them because of an illness or a disability. Traditionally, we have developed separate worlds in order to meet people's needs. For example, separate workshops, education groups and living accommodation for people with mental health needs, dementia or any type of disability have kept people out of the mainstream of society. Older people have been separated with clubs, day centres and residential accommodation on the assumption that separate is best. But increasingly, we have come to see that separate is not equal, and we should have an inclusive society that everyone can enjoy.

Now, we are asking different questions about how we organise society. We do not ask, 'What is wrong with this person that means they cannot use the leisure centre or the cinema?' Instead we ask, 'What is wrong with the cinema or the leisure centre if people with disabilities can't use it?'

Inclusive practice is about providing the support that people want in order to live their lives as fully as possible. Examples of inclusive practice are:

- changing the physical shape and colour of buildings to reduce confusion for people with dementia

- providing plenty of spaces where people with dementia can walk or pace if they want to

- having large, clear signs to provide information

- ensuring that systems and processes for obtaining support are easy to use, with clear, simple choices and support if needed.

Overall, practising in an inclusive way means constantly asking 'What changes need to happen so that this person can participate?' and then doing whatever is within your area of responsibility to make those changes happen. In order for anyone to be included in society, we have to make the necessary changes for it to be possible.

Working with carers

As a carer of a loved family member, it is not always easy to remember that the person you are caring for should be able to make choices and decisions for themselves. Very often, people think that if someone was capable of making decisions, they would not need to be looked after. It is important that the underlying principles about rights and choices are explained to carers so that they can also support the person to take more control.

Some carers can see that this approach is right following an explanation and discussion, while others may feel more reassured if they have the opportunity to see how it works in action and may be interested to look at some case studies, or even talk to other carers who are also supporting relatives with dementia.

Just as each person with dementia has a unique experience, carers also are unique in how they respond to the demands of caring and consider new information and approaches.

Getting ready for assessment

DEM 310 is a knowledge unit, so each of the learning outcomes requires you to show your assessor that you have understood the learning. Your assessor may ask you to produce a written assignment or project, or to prepare a presentation or a computer-based exercise. Sometimes, assessors will check your understanding through a professional discussion where you will answer questions that demonstrate that you understand all the learning.

This unit is all about equality, diversity and inclusion, so you will have to show that you understand why these matter and how they affect the way services for people with dementia are delivered. Your assessor will want to see that you have understood how inclusive working makes dementia services more accessible. They will also want to see that you have understood how to recognise the diversity of people's individual and unique needs.

Person-centred working is also a key part of this unit, and you may be able to use some of the assessment evidence from other units to meet this learning outcome.

Some of the assessment criteria ask for specific things. For example, when you are asked to explain, do not

simply list or describe; use words such as 'because', 'as a result of', 'so that', 'in order to'. If you are explaining something you must show that you understand the reasons for it.

DEM 313 is a competence unit that requires knowledge and demonstration of skills. You will need to demonstrate in a workplace setting that you are able to work in a person-centred way with people and their carers and families. You must show that you have found out as much as possible about the person you are supporting and that you know how their history influences their present. Your assessor will want to see that you have used a life history to help you to meet a person's needs.

You will also need to show that you can support people from a range of ethnic and cultural backgrounds and that you understand how dementia can be different for people who are younger or who have a learning disability.

You may be able to use some of the assessment evidence, particularly regarding person-centred working, from other units.

Further reading and research

- www.alzheimers.org.uk (Alzheimer's Society: information about attitudes towards dementia).
- www.dh.gov.uk/en/Publicationsandstatistics/Publications/PublicationsPolicyAndGuidance/DH_094058 (Department of Health: Living well with dementia: A National Dementia Strategy).
- www.ncpc.org.uk (National Council for Palliative Care: information about providing high-quality end-of-life care).
- www.scie.org.uk (Social Care Institute for Excellence: information about attitudes towards dementia).

DEM 304

Enable rights and choices for people with dementia whilst minimising risks

When you are working with people with dementia, you need to balance a person's rights and choices against risks to their safety and that of others. People have rights regardless of the stage of their dementia, but they also have a right to be protected from serious harm. Sometimes this may mean that their freedoms have to be limited to avoid serious risk. These are difficult balances to achieve and you will need to understand the issues involved in the decisions you will have to make. This will help you to take the best possible action for people with dementia to exercise their rights and make choices about their lives without coming to serious harm.

In this unit you will learn about:

■ key legislation and agreed ways of working that support the fulfilment of rights and choices of people with dementia whilst minimising risk of harm
■ how to maximise the rights and choices of people with dementia
■ how to involve carers and others in supporting people with dementia
■ how to maintain the privacy, dignity and respect of people with dementia whilst promoting rights and choices.

1: Legislation and ways of working that balance rights and choices and minimise risks

1.1 The impact of key legislation

Basic human rights

In 1949 the United Nations Universal Declaration of Human Rights identified a set of basic rights that everyone should have. The Declaration sets out to promote and encourage acceptance of personal, **civil**, political, economic, social and cultural rights. These rights are only limited by the need to respect the rights and freedoms of others and the needs of morality, public order and general welfare. There are 30 articles in the Declaration and they cover all aspects of rights. You can find out more about the detail of these rights by visiting the United Nations website – see the Further reading and research section at the end of this chapter.

> **Key terms**
>
> **Civil** – relating to ordinary citizens and their concerns.
>
> **Public body** – an organisation whose work is part of the process is government, but which is not a government department.

For many people throughout the world, these are rights they can only hope for, and not rights they currently enjoy. The United Nations has the office of the High Commission for Human Rights (OHCHR) that works to promote the worldwide acceptance of these basic rights and to identify abuses and violations of human rights throughout the world. These basic human rights apply to everyone, regardless of their position in life, their circumstances or the way in which they are affected by any medical condition, including dementia. These rights form the basis of human rights legislation in the UK and Europe.

Human Rights Act 1998

In the UK human rights are protected by the Human Rights Act 1998. Under this Act, residents of the United Kingdom (this Act applies in England, Scotland, Wales and Northern Ireland) are entitled to seek help from the UK courts if they believe that their human rights have been infringed by any **public body**. If people feel that they have not had justice from the UK courts, they can take their case to the European Court of Human Rights, which sits in Strasbourg and is the highest court for human rights in Europe.

The Human Rights Act applies to public bodies and to organisations that work on behalf of public bodies.

The definition of a public body covers many different bodies, including:

- government departments
- local authorities
- police
- benefits agencies
- the courts.

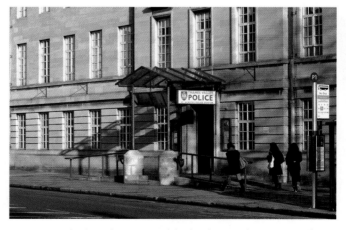

Have you dealt with many public bodies in the course of your work?

It also includes organisations that carry out any 'public function'. The Act does not identify precisely what it means by a public function, but it is generally taken to mean:

- when an organisation performs or operates in the public domain as part of a **statutory** system (e.g. social services, police, courts, prisons)
- when it performs a duty that is of public significance
- when the rights or obligations of individuals are affected by the performance of the duty
- when a body is non-statutory but is established under the authority of government or local government (e.g. agencies contracted to deliver services)
- when a body performs functions that the government or local government would otherwise perform
- when an individual may have some legitimate expectation in performance of the duty (e.g. in receiving healthcare).

Key term

Statutory – required, permitted or created by law.

Table 5.1: Organisations subject to the Human Rights Act 1998

Residential homes or nursing homes	These perform functions which would otherwise be performed by a local authority.
Charities	
Voluntary organisations	
Public services	These include the privatised utilities, such as gas, electric and water companies, which perform duties of public significance.

Within the health and care sector there are many organisations whose work is covered by the Human Rights Act. For example:

- Meals services, which are to a great extent provided by the voluntary sector, are likely to be seen as fulfilling part of the statutory duties of the local authority. Therefore, they have to ensure that they are not restricting anyone's human rights, for example, by failing to provide meals that meet somebody's religious dietary requirements.
- Domiciliary care services, many of which are run by the private sector, also have to ensure that their services

are provided within the requirements of the Act. They have to ensure that all the carers are fully aware of the implications of the Act in their day-to-day work.

It is likely that anyone who works in health or care will be working within the provisions of the Human Rights Act. This Act is all about respecting, promoting and fostering the rights of individual people throughout all the functions of the organisation, whether it is a public body or an organisation that is carrying out the role of a public body. The rights protected under the Act are:

1 **The right to life.** Public bodies must not cause the death of any person and they have a positive obligation to protect life. The Act specifies a limited number of circumstances where it is not a contravention of the Act to take someone's life. But this only applies where the force used is no more than absolutely necessary, in situations such as defending a person from attack or making a lawful arrest.

2 **The right to freedom from torture and inhuman or degrading treatment or punishment.** Torture is identified as the most serious kind of ill-treatment. Inhuman or degrading treatment is less severe than torture. It includes physical assaults, inhuman detention conditions and corporal punishment, and relates to both mental and physical suffering. One of the factors that is taken into account under this right is the severity and duration of the torture, degrading treatment or punishment and the vulnerability of the victim. This is very relevant for people with dementia and for any vulnerable groups. There have been many reported cases of abuse in residential establishments and by professional carers in positions of power.

3 **The right to freedom from slavery, servitude and forced or compulsory labour.** Slavery means that a person is owned like a piece of property. Servitude is when a person is not owned by someone else but is in enforced service and is unable to leave. There are some exceptions to this right, for example, work that is carried out as part of a prison sentence.

4 **The right to liberty and security of person.** People have the right not to be arrested or detained, except when the detention is authorised by law. This part of the Act does not just apply to police arrests but covers all aspects of detention, including for medical or psychiatric reasons. There are clearly defined circumstances in which people can be detained, such as after conviction by a court or where there are sufficient grounds to believe that they may have committed a crime.

5   **The right to a fair and public trial within a reasonable time.** This right covers all criminal and most civil cases, as well as **tribunals** and some internal hearings (within an organisation). People have the right to be presumed innocent until proven guilty and to be given adequate time and facilities to prepare their defence. The Act gives everyone a right to a trial in public so that justice can never be carried out behind closed doors.

6   **The right to freedom from retrospective criminal law and no punishment without law.** This right means that people cannot be convicted of an act that was not a criminal offence at the time it was committed, nor can they face a punishment which was not in place when the act happened.

7   **The right to respect for private and family life, home and correspondence.** This part of the Human Rights Act protects many areas of people's lives. Public bodies may only interfere in someone's private life when they have the legal authority to do so. This right covers matters such as the disclosure of private information, monitoring of telephone calls and email, and carrying out searches. It imposes restrictions on entering a person's home. It also covers issues such as the right of families to live together and the right not to suffer from environmental hazards.

8   **The right to freedom of thought, conscience and religion.** Under this right people can hold whatever thoughts, ethical views and religious beliefs that they wish. They are guaranteed the right to practise their religion or belief in worship, teaching, practice and observance.

9   **The right to freedom of expression.** Freedom of expression includes what is said in conversation or speeches, what is published in books, articles or leaflets, what is broadcast and what is presented as art or placed on the Internet – in fact, any means of communication.

10 **The right to freedom of assembly and association.** This includes the right of people to demonstrate peacefully and to join, or choose not to join, trade unions.

11 **The right to marry and found a family.** This part of the Act is particularly relevant to rules and policies concerning adoption and fostering. Public bodies have to ensure that their policies in this area are not contravening the Act, for example, policies to do with the age or race of applicants to become adoptive parents.

12 **The prohibition of discrimination in the enjoyment of convention rights.** The Act recognises that not all differences in treatment are discriminatory. Those that are discriminatory are defined as having no objective or reasonable justification. For example, if a registry office provided information about how to undertake a civil marriage in English only, this could affect the human rights of someone who was unable to speak English and was therefore unable to access the information they need. This could be said to be denying them the means to exercise their human right to marry. It would probably be viewed as discriminatory because there is no objective or reasonable justification for failing to provide information in other languages. Another example is if a young person was excluded from school and therefore unable to exercise their human right to receive an education. If it could be proved they were excluded because of their disruptive behaviour and not because of race, socioeconomic circumstances or other type of discrimination, then this would not be discriminatory.

13 **The right to peaceful enjoyment of possessions and protection of property.** The Act defines many possessions as property; not just things like houses and cars, but also shares, licences and **goodwill**. In some circumstances the right to engage in a profession can be regarded as a property right. Under the Act no one can be deprived of their property, except where the action is permitted by law.

14 **The right to access an education.** The right of access to education must be balanced against the resources available. This right must be considered when deciding whether to exclude a disruptive pupil from school, and when providing education for children with special needs.

15 **The right to free elections.** Elections must be free and fair and be held at reasonable intervals. This right covers issues of participation and access, including making sure that people with disabilities or those who are ill are still able to participate.

16 **The right not to be subjected to the death penalty.** This provision confirms the abolition of the death penalty.

Key terms

Tribunal – a special court convened by government to inquire into a specific matter.

Goodwill – the established reputation of a business regarded as an asset.

These rights are given in general terms, and they can be interpreted for individuals. Within social care, making sure that people's rights are protected is a key part of your professional role.

When someone has dementia, it is sometimes easy for people to forget that they also have the same human rights as everyone else. Just because someone is not always able to defend their rights or to make sure that the law is protecting them does not mean that their rights are any less important or that they can be ignored.

The Human Rights Act raises awareness of how human rights can be affected by the way that public services are delivered and interpreted, and clarifies exactly what the responsibilities of government and people delivering services are. Prior to the Act, people may have assumed that they had those rights, but it was only after the Act was passed that they became legally enforceable.

What does the Human Rights Act mean in practice at work?

Under the Human Rights Act all other legislation must be read, understood and used in a way that is compatible with the requirements of the Human Rights Act. You are required to make every effort to interpret the legislation that you work with so that it is compatible with the Human Rights Act. This means that if there are two possible interpretations of the provision under another act (such as the Mental Health Act, the Children Act or the Community Care Act), it is the interpretation that is compatible with the Human Rights Act that you must follow.

Government guidance states that all public bodies have a positive obligation to ensure that respect for human rights is at the core of their day-to-day work. This guidance covers all aspects of an organisation's activities, including:

- drafting rules and regulations and policies
- internal staff and personnel issues
- administration
- decision making
- implementing policy and working with members of the public.

Equality Act

The Equality Act 2010 protects the rights of individuals and provides equality of opportunity. It replaces many previous acts, including:

- most of the provisions of the Disability Discrimination Acts 1995 and 2005

- the Equal Pay Act 1970
- the Sex Discrimination Act 1975
- the Race Relations Act 1976
- the Special Educational Needs and Disability Act 2001
- the Racial and Religious Hatred Act 2006
- the Equality Act 2006.

The Equality Act now protects different groups of people under just one act. There are nine 'protected grounds' where the Act requires there to be equality: age, disability, gender, race, religion and belief, pregnancy and maternity, marriage and civil partnership, sexual orientation and gender reassignment.

Broadly, the Act covers:

- the basic framework of protection against direct and indirect discrimination, harassment and victimisation in services and public functions, premises, work, education, associations and transport
- changing the definition of gender reassignment, by removing the requirement for medical supervision
- levelling up protection for people discriminated against because they are perceived to have, or are associated with someone who has, a **protected characteristic**, so providing new protection for people like carers
- clearer protection for breastfeeding mothers
- applying the European definition of indirect discrimination to all protected characteristics
- extending protection from indirect discrimination to disability
- introducing a new concept of 'discrimination arising from disability', to replace protection under previous legislation lost as a result of a legal judgement
- where people are disadvantaged by discrimination, they will be able to claim
- all employers have a duty to make reasonable adjustments for disabled people
- extending protection from third party harassment to all protected characteristics

> **Key term**
>
> **Protected characteristic** – these include age, disability, gender reassignment, marriage and civil partnership, pregnancy and maternity, race, religion and belief, sex and sexual orientation.

- making it more difficult for disabled people to be unfairly screened out when applying for jobs, by restricting the circumstances in which employers can ask job applicants questions about disability or health
- allowing hypothetical ways of comparing for direct gender pay discrimination
- making pay secrecy clauses unenforceable
- extending protection in private clubs to sex, religion or belief, pregnancy and maternity, and gender reassignment
- introducing new powers for employment tribunals to make recommendations that benefit the wider workforce
- harmonising provisions allowing voluntary positive action.

How does the Equality Act protect people with dementia?

Although not all of the Equality Act will be relevant for everyone with dementia, it will be relevant for younger people in the early stages of dementia who may wish to continue working for as long as possible in order to retain their independence. This Act ensures that employers must make reasonable adjustments to enable them to do their job and cannot discriminate against them because of their condition. It also protects people in their social and leisure activities and requires that places where there is public access must make it possible for people with dementia to use the facilities.

Under the Act, a person is defined as having a disability if:

- they have a physical or mental impairment
- the impairment has a substantial and long-term adverse effect on their ability to perform normal day-to-day activities.

For the purposes of the Act, these words have the following meanings:

- 'substantial' means more than minor or trivial
- 'long-term' means that the effect of the impairment has lasted or is likely to last for at least 12 months
- 'normal day-to-day activities' include everyday things like eating, washing, walking and going shopping.

These definitions are important because it is very clear that most people with dementia are covered by the provisions of the Act and are protected from discrimination.

The Equality and Human Rights Commission has a statutory remit to promote and monitor human rights in the UK. The Commission protects and enforces equality across the nine 'protected grounds' under the Act.

Activity 1

- Find out about the work of the Equality and Human Rights Commission in the UK and how it applies to people with dementia.
- Research any issues that have been taken up by the Commission that have implications for people with dementia. For example, a recent investigation into home care found that older people were having their human rights breached. See what else you can find.

Mental Capacity Act 2005

The Mental Capacity Act (MCA) sets out a framework for supporting people to make decisions, and lays out the ways in which people can be supported. The Act applies to England and Wales. Scotland has similar provision in the Adults with Incapacity (Scotland) Act (AIA).

The MCA is underpinned by five key principles:

1 A presumption of capacity: Every adult has the right to make their own decisions and must be assumed to have capacity to do so unless it is proved otherwise.

2 The right for individuals to be supported to make their own decisions: People must be given all appropriate help, including advocates and support workers, before anyone concludes that they cannot make their own decisions.

3 Individuals must retain the right to make what might be seen as eccentric or unwise decisions: Just because someone decides to do something that may seem foolish or risky, it does not mean that they are incapable of making decisions. After all, everyone does silly things sometimes.

4 Best interests: Anything done for or on behalf of people without capacity must be in their best interests.

5 Least restrictive intervention: Anything done for or on behalf of people without capacity should be the least restrictive of their basic rights and freedoms.

The Act sets out clearly how to establish whether someone is incapable of taking a decision, using a 'capacity test' (see below). This test can only be applied in relation to a particular decision. No one can be deemed 'incapable' in general simply because of a medical condition or diagnosis.

The Act introduced a new criminal offence of ill-treatment or neglect of a person who lacks capacity. A person found guilty of such an offence may be liable to imprisonment for a term of up to five years.

How the Mental Capacity Act applies to people with dementia

This Act is very important for people with dementia. Traditionally, there has been an assumption that people who have dementia have no capacity to make decisions. There was no legislation to protect them from having decisions made about their lives without their involvement or agreement. Since the implementation of the MCA and AIA (Scotland), people must now have the opportunity to consider and make decisions for themselves wherever possible.

It is also an important principle that incapacity is related to a specific instance. It can never be assumed that, because someone has dementia, they cannot make any decisions. Someone may be incapable of deciding when to take their medication because they have no idea of time, but that does not mean that they cannot refuse to sell their home because they may be very clear that this is something they do not want to do. It is the decision-making process, and the person's ability to go through the process, that is looked at under the Act, not the outcome of the decisions a person makes.

The assessment of capacity is the responsibility of the person who wants a decision to be made. For example, if the question is about medical consent, the health professional concerned needs to make the assessment. If it is about moving into residential care, then it would be the social worker. In the case of major decisions, or where is there is doubt, the professional concerned will usually refer to a psychiatrist or psychologist for a second opinion.

Capacity test

The capacity test looks at the functions of decision making. The Act states that a person lacks capacity regarding a decision if there is 'an impairment of, or a disturbance in the functioning of, the mind or brain'. The assessment aims to find out whether, at the time the decision needs to be taken, the person is unable to do one or more of the following:

- understand the information relevant to the decision
- retain the information relevant to the decision
- use and weigh the information to arrive at a decision
- communicate the decision (by any means).

To be judged to have capacity, people must be able to do all of the parts of the test.

Adults with Incapacity (Scotland) Act

The Adults with Incapacity (Scotland) Act is very similar to the Mental Capacity Act – it has the same criteria for judging capacity and shares similar principles with the MCA.

Under this Act, as for the Mental Capacity Act, anyone authorised to make decisions on behalf of someone with impaired capacity must apply the following principles:

- **Benefit:** Any action or decision taken must benefit the person and only be taken when that benefit cannot reasonably be achieved without it.
- **Least restrictive option:** Any action or decision taken should be the minimum necessary to achieve the purpose. It should be the option that restricts the person's freedom as little as possible.
- **Take account of the wishes of the person:** In deciding if an action or decision is to be made, account must be taken of the present and past wishes and feelings of the person. Some people may not be capable of making a particular decision, but will be able to express their wishes and feelings clearly. The person must be offered help to communicate their views. This might mean using memory aids, pictures, non-verbal communication, a speech and language therapist or support from an independent advocate.
- **Consultation with relevant others:** The Act lists the people who should be consulted whenever practicable and reasonable. It includes the person's primary carer, nearest relative, named person, attorney or guardian (if there is one).
- **Encourage the person to use existing skills and develop new skills.**

In Scotland if someone lacks the capacity to make a decision, then a Welfare Guardian will be appointed. This can be a relative, a friend or a social worker.

Reflect

Think about a decision you have made. Look at each of the four parts of the capacity test. Make notes about how you made your decision and link your process to each of the parts of the capacity assessment. Can you see how you followed the process of reaching a decision?

For example, you might have been deciding to get a new job, buy a new computer or move house. Any of those decisions would involve you going through a process before finally deciding. Think about how decisions are made and how the process applies to the people you support.

Deprivation of Liberty Safeguards (DoLS)

Safeguards for the MCA were introduced in 2009, following a court case about a young man who was detained in hospital without giving, or refusing, his consent. He lacked the capacity to willingly consent or refuse to be in hospital. In the light of this case, the Deprivation of Liberty Safeguards (DoLS) were introduced. These require that assessments are carried out before anyone can be detained in a hospital, a residential care home or any other facility.

The concept of deprivation of liberty can cover many different situations. Courts have been involved in several different cases, including:

- a patient being restrained in order to admit them to hospital
- medication being given against a person's will
- staff having complete control over a patient's care or movements for a long period
- staff making all decisions about a patient, including choices about assessments, treatment and visitors
- staff deciding whether a patient can be released into the care of others or to live elsewhere
- staff refusing to discharge a person into the care of others
- staff restricting a person's access to their friends or family.

If a facility wishes to use any form of restraint, there are very strict procedures to be followed. A residential care facility must contact social services, who will arrange for a specially trained 'Best Interests Assessor' to decide if the deprivation of liberty is justified. There are clear guidelines for the Assessor to follow, and a set of criteria that the person must meet. If the Assessor is satisfied, then they will agree to an authorisation for that person. There must also be agreement from a 'Mental Health Assessor', who must be a doctor (usually a psychiatrist or geriatrician). An authorisation is made for the shortest possible time, but can be for up to a year.

People who have their liberty restricted must have a 'relevant person's representative' (RPR). Usually this will be a family member or friend, but where this is not possible, they will have the services of an Independent Mental Capacity Advocate (IMCA). The role of the RPR is to ensure that the person's rights are respected and that they, as far as possible, understand about how their liberty is being restricted. All of those involved with the person are required to ensure that the RPR has all the information about the decision and the ongoing support of the person.

Activity 2

Find out about how the DoLS applies in your workplace. Check if any authorisations have been applied for and what the circumstances were. Find out about the reasons for the decision to seek DoLS authorisation. Make notes about the differences or similarities between the reasons for the request and the circumstances of the people concerned.

Mental Health Act 2007

The Mental Health Act 2007 made some changes to the Mental Health Act 1983. People with dementia can be detained in a hospital under the Mental Health Act if they are considered to be behaving in a way that causes a danger to themselves or others. The 2007 Act allows people to have a guardian appointed to make decisions on their behalf, and to ensure that they comply with any requirements in relation to their health. A guardian can decide where someone has to live and make sure that they attend appointments.

One of the new provisions in the Act is that 'nearest relative' can now include a civil partner, and anyone who is detained under the Mental Health Act can challenge the person who is considered to be their nearest relative. For example, someone may have a son whom they have not seen for a long time, but he is legally the nearest relative; they may also have a niece who visits them daily. Previously, it would not have been possible for the niece to have been designated as the nearest relative, but now the person can request it.

Anyone who is detained in hospital under the Mental Health Act can have access to an Independent Mental Health Advocate (IMCA) who can explain their rights.

Some important terms used in legislation

Mental disorder

Mental disorder is the term used in the Mental Health Act. Dementia is considered to be a mental disorder and therefore the Act can apply to people with dementia.

Approved Mental Health Practitioner

An Approved Mental Health Practitioner is a professional who is involved in decisions about whether someone is detained under the Act. They are also involved in decisions about appointing a guardian. They are usually a social worker, but can be another mental health professional (such as a community psychiatric nurse) who is trained and approved to perform this role.

Nearest relative

The nearest relative looks after the interests of the person concerned. There is a list that is followed and the person closest to the top of the list is considered to be the nearest relative:

- husband, wife or civil partner
- son or daughter
- father or mother
- brother or sister
- grandparent
- grandchild
- uncle or aunt
- nephew or niece
- someone (not a relative) the person has lived with for at least the last five years.

The nearest relative can request that someone is detained in hospital, object to a guardian, discharge the person from hospital and apply to a tribunal for someone to be discharged.

A court can change the designated nearest relative under certain circumstances if they have a request from a healthcare professional or the person themselves. This could be done if it is considered that the nearest relative is trying to discharge someone without sufficient regard for their welfare or the welfare of others, unreasonably objecting to a guardianship order or detention for treatment, or being unable to fulfil their role due to illness.

Responsible clinician

The responsible clinician is the health professional in charge of the person's care in the hospital. This is normally a doctor, but it can be another health professional such as a psychologist, social worker, mental health nurse or occupational therapist who has been approved to perform this role.

Independent Mental Health Advocate

An Independent Mental Health Advocate is someone who can explain a person's rights and provide information and advice about how to challenge a section decision to compulsorily detain someone in hospital. Advocates have access to the person's medical records and operate independently from the hospital.

Managing risks

There are always risks involved in appointing people to the workforce that supports vulnerable groups, such as people with dementia. Some people may try to take advantage of people with dementia for personal gain; others may want to be in a position of power and could exploit or harm those people whom they should be supporting.

There are organisations responsible for checking the suitability of people to work in social care. In England, Wales and Northern Ireland this is done by the Independent Safeguarding Authority (ISA), which maintains the list of people barred from working with children and young people and also the list of those barred from working with vulnerable adults. In Scotland the Protecting Vulnerable Groups (PVG) scheme has the same lists, which are maintained by Disclosure Scotland. The same organisation is also responsible for identifying any criminal records of people who want to work with any vulnerable groups. In Northern Ireland these checks are carried out by Access NI and in England and Wales by the Criminal Records Bureau (CRB).

Changes in how these risks are managed recently took place under the Protection of Freedoms Act 2011, which became law in May 2012. This Act will combine the ISA and CRB into one organisation, called the Disclosure and Barring Service (DBS). This is planned for December 2012 and will provide a system of 'portable' criminal records checks and reduce the number of people who have to be subject to checks.

1.2 Ways of working

Wherever you work, there will be policies and procedures about how to make sure that people's rights are protected and that you are working within the relevant legislation. If you are working as a personal assistant directly employed by someone with dementia, you are an example of how that person is exercising their rights and choice. By choosing to employ someone directly, they are maintaining control over how and when their support is delivered. However, it is still your responsibility to carry out your **duty of care** and to make sure that your actions are promoting your employer's rights and that you are working within the law and national guidelines.

> **Key term**
>
> **Duty of care** – a legal obligation to do everything you can to keep those in your care safe from harm.

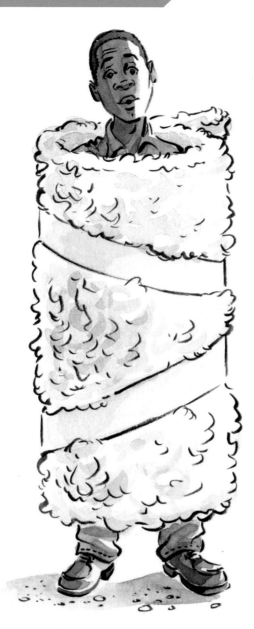

Figure 5.1: Carrying out your duty of care does not mean wrapping people in cotton wool

Having codes of practice is important; working with people who have dementia involves working with some of the most vulnerable people in society. They have a right to expect a certain standard of work and a certain standard of moral and ethical behaviour.

In order to work in social work anywhere in the UK and in social care in some parts (soon to be all) of the UK, there is a requirement to be registered. This means having, or working towards, a certain minimum level of qualification and agreeing to work within the Code of Practice, which sets out the behaviour that is required. Employers have to ensure that everyone who works for them is registered and eligible to work in social work or social care. At the moment only social care practitioners in Scotland and Wales are registered, but England and Northern Ireland will be following in the near future. In any event, abiding by the Codes of Practice is a good way of making sure that your practice is following ethical and professional guidelines.

Codes of practice

The regulatory bodies in the UK have codes of practice both for employers in the social care field and for the social care workforce. The General Social Care Council in England, the Scottish Social Services Council, the Care Council Wales and the Northern Ireland Social Services Council have similar codes covering key areas of practice. These require the workforce to do the following.

- Protect the rights and promote the interests of individuals and carers. This includes respect for individuality and support for individuals to control their own lives, and respect for and maintenance of equal opportunities, diversity, dignity and privacy.

- Establish and maintain the trust and confidence of individuals and carers. This means not abusing, neglecting or exploiting individuals or colleagues, or forming inappropriate personal relationships, not discriminating or condoning discrimination, or placing oneself or others at unnecessary risk, and not abusing the trust of others in relation to confidentiality

- Uphold public trust and confidence in social care services. This includes maintaining confidentiality, using effective communication, honouring commitments and agreements, declaring conflicts of interest and adhering to policies about accepting gifts.

- Promote the independence of individuals while protecting them from danger or harm. This means recognising the right to take risks, following risk assessment policies, minimising risks and ensuring others are informed about risk assessments.

If you are employed by an organisation, there will be policies and processes in place to make sure that people are able to exercise their right to make choices about how they live and what they do. These are rights that do not have the force of law, but which are enforceable within social care and are designed to improve the quality of services that people receive.

Your professional responsibility is to act within the Code of Practice of the regulator for the UK country in which you work. This lays out the duties and expectations for everyone who works in the sector.

- Respect the rights of individuals while seeking to ensure that their behaviour does not harm themselves or other people. This includes maintenance of rights, challenging and reporting dangerous, abusive, discriminatory or exploitative behaviour, following safe practice, reporting resource problems, reporting unsafe practice of colleagues, following health and safety regulations, helping individuals to make complaints and using power responsibly.

- Be accountable for the quality of one's work and take responsibility for maintaining and improving your knowledge and skills. This means meeting standards, maintaining appropriate records and informing employers of personal difficulties.

National Minimum Standards

Each of the countries of the UK has a body that is responsible for inspecting all social care facilities to make sure that they are complying with National Minimum Standards. These bodies are:

- the Care Quality Commission in England
- the Care Inspectorate in Scotland
- the Care and Social Services Inspectorate in Wales
- the Regulation and Quality Improvement Authority in Northern Ireland.

Each of them uses a series of National Minimum Standards in order to inspect the quality of care. There are different sets of standards for different types of services. For example, there are separate standards for care homes for older people and for younger adults, for children's homes and for fostering services. The standards documents provide a detailed set of definitions that outline the minimum quality of care that an individual may expect. All of the organisations also provide user-friendly information for people who are using the services about the levels of service that they can expect to receive.

Standards are important because they tell people what is the very least that they can reasonably expect from someone providing their support. Of course, most providers will aim to deliver higher-quality services, but they must comply with the minimum standards. If people know what is expected of a provider, then they have a basis on which to make a complaint if the service fails to meet the expected quality.

Knowing about entitlements and expectations is an essential part of being able to protect rights. If people do not know what should be available, it is much harder for them to know if their rights are being protected. National Minimum Standards are also useful for you, as a professional, to know what should be being delivered in your work setting.

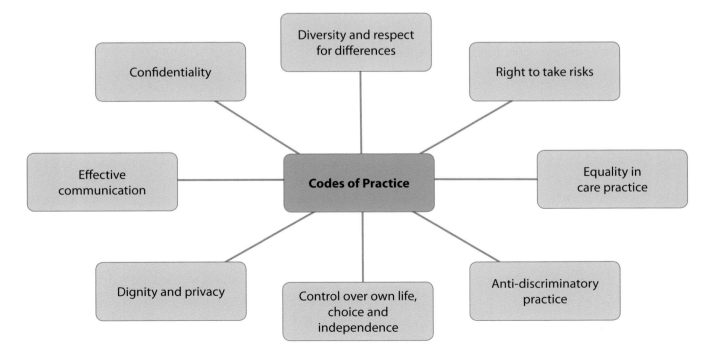

Figure 5.2: Rights covered by the Codes of Practice

Rights and responsibilities

Rights also involve responsibilities. Everyone has the responsibility not to infringe the rights of other people. Some responsibilities that are linked to the rights in Figure 5.2 are set out in Table 5.2. These responsibilities apply to you and to the people you support. Understanding this balance is important; it is easy to forget that sometimes one person exercising their rights may restrict the rights of others. For example, someone may claim the right of free speech to make racist comments about people from other ethnic groups. Clearly this is unacceptable because it infringes other people's fundamental right to be respected and valued as individuals, and it is racist, discriminatory and illegal.

It is important to understand that the right to 'free speech' does not mean that people can say whatever they like. Speech is only 'free' as long as it does not infringe the rights of others by being discriminatory, slanderous or inciting hatred.

One person may believe that they have a right to enjoyment of their music at whatever volume they want to play it – but this is not true if it affects the rights of others to enjoy peace and quiet. In a group living situation, such conflicts between rights and responsibilities can be difficult to resolve and you may have to deal with issues like this frequently.

Rights and responsibilities are always finely balanced. Some examples are given in Table 5.2.

1.3 Sharing information

Every organisation will have policies on confidentiality and the disclosure of information. You must be sure that you know what both these policies are in your workplace.

Confidentiality and disclosing information

The basic rule is that all information an individual gives, or that is given on their behalf, to an organisation is confidential and cannot be disclosed to anyone without the consent of the individual. You will need to support people in contributing to and understanding records and reports concerning them, and ensure they understand how the rules of confidentiality affect them. This can be difficult when people have dementia and may have difficulty in processing and retaining information. It is important to reassure people that their information

Table 5.2: Examples of how rights also involve responsibilities

Right	Responsibility
Diversity and the right to be different	Respect for diversity in others
Equality and freedom from discrimination	Respect for the equality of others and valuing members of other social groups
Control over own life, choice and independence	Making choices that respect others' independence, choices and lifestyles
Freedom to choose lifestyle, self-presentation, diet and routine	Considering the consequences of choices for the person and others around them
Dignity and privacy	Respect for the dignity and privacy of others
To be valued as an individual	Respect for the identity needs of others
Confidentiality	Respect for the confidentiality of others
To be safe and secure	To behave in a way that does not threaten or abuse the physical or emotional safety and security of others
To take risks, including taking risks as a matter of choice, in order to maintain the individual's own identity or perceived well-being	Not to expose oneself or others to unacceptable risks, and be willing to negotiate about the impact of risk on others

is confidential and you may have to repeat this regularly and provide people with the information in the way that works best for them.

In many cases, passing on information is routine and related to the care of the person concerned. For example, medical information may be passed on to a hospital, residential home or private care agency. However, this is only with the agreement of the person concerned. Even if they have chosen to commission a particular service, you must still make it clear that information will have to be shared. Do not assume that the person will realise this, and do not assume that they will not object. Always ask, for example, by saying: 'So now that you've chosen the agency, you do realise that we'll have to pass on the information in your records? Are you OK about this?'

But it is essential that only information that is required for the purpose is passed on. For example, it is not necessary to tell the dentist that Mrs Winton's son, who is her next of kin, is currently serving a prison sentence. However, if Mrs Winton became seriously ill and the hospital wanted to contact her next of kin, you would need to pass that information on. The dentist would, however, need to know that Mrs Winton's teeth had been getting loose due to her Alzheimer's-related weight loss and that she has been having a very sore mouth as a result.

When is it right to share information?

People have a right to confidentiality, but also a responsibility in relation to the rights of others. Confidentiality often has to be kept within boundaries and the rights of others have to be balanced with the person's rights. For example, a support worker may have to tell their manager something learned in confidence, or they may have to seek medical assistance for someone.

Table 5.3 gives some examples of situations in which you have to pass on information, because keeping it to yourself could result in harm to the person you are supporting, to someone else or to yourself.

In all of the situations given in Table 5.3, you must only share the information with a manager in order to decide what action to take. You must not share this information any further without consultation with senior colleagues.

If you are directly employed as a personal assistant and are concerned about the well-being of your employer, you may have to pass on information to the relevant organisation: social services, doctor or police. These are not easy decisions to make and you will have to be very clear about why you think that someone is not able to make decisions that are in their own best interests. The reason may be that they are ill or confused, or because they are afraid of someone else. The Mental Capacity Act 2005 lays down very strict criteria for deciding whether a person can make a decision (see page 91), so this is not something to be decided by an individual worker or manager. The procedures must be followed in these circumstances.

In the situation where a person is afraid of someone, but does have capacity to make a decision, the only thing you can do is to try to persuade them to agree to take action. In Scotland there are powers that enable

Table 5.3: Situations in which you might have to pass on information

Situation	Example
There is a significant risk of harm to someone.	An older person tells you that she switches off the heating as soon as there is no one in the house, in order to save money. She asks you not to tell anyone because her daughter will make a fuss. She may be at risk of harm from the cold.
A person is in danger of being abused.	A man explains that his son takes his money, but asks you not to tell anyone because his son will be angry and the man is frightened of him. He is experiencing financial abuse.
There is a significant risk of harm to others.	A person lives in a terraced house piled high with newspapers and rubbish. He tells you that he lights fires in the hearth with some of the old newspapers. He begs you not to tell anyone because he is terrified that 'they' will make him move out of his home. There is a serious risk of fire, not only in his house, but also of it spreading to other houses in the street.
There is a risk to the support worker's health or well-being.	A person is very aggressive and becoming violent, placing you at risk. You know that he can be calm at times and usually responds well to you, but recently he has been becoming more and more aggressive.

social workers to intervene, but not in the rest of the UK. If someone is an adult with capacity, they are able to make the decision not to share information or to make a complaint or report to the police.

Doing it well

Decisions about breaking confidentiality are about balancing the risks – ask yourself: 'Are the risks of the distress caused by my breaking confidentiality greater than the risks posed to a person's health and well-being by the circumstances?'

Making a decision that you know could damage a relationship you have built up with someone over a period of time is always hard to do. This is particularly difficult when you work with people who have dementia. The progressive nature of dementia means that you will frequently have to re-assess a person's capacity to make decisions and to review the risks posed by any situation. If at all possible, discuss the circumstances with a manager or senior colleague before deciding on action.

Remember that the well-being of the person you are supporting is always the deciding factor.

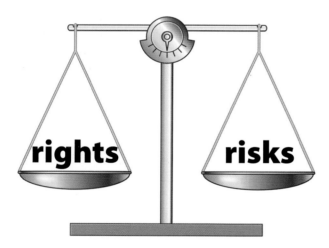

Figure 5.3: Experience will help with balancing rights and risks

Confidentiality and the need to know

Good practice involves asking people whether you can let other people know things about their situation. Whatever you know should be kept private unless the person concerned tells you that it is acceptable to share the information. Sometimes information can be passed

on when others have a need to know it. Some examples of people who have a 'need to know' are:

- managers – they may need to help make decisions which affect the person
- colleagues – they may be working with the same person
- other professionals – they may also be working with the person and need to be kept up to date.

However, information should always be shared with the knowledge and consent of the person concerned. You must always explain that you will be passing on information and what the information is, so that people do not imagine that you will be telling others everything about them. When people have a need to know, they only need to know enough to do their job.

When information is passed on to other professionals, it should be on the understanding that they keep it confidential. It is important to check that people asking for information are who they say they are. If you answer the telephone and the caller says they are a social worker or other professional, you should explain that you must call back before giving any information. Phoning back enables you to be sure that you are talking to someone at a particular number or within a particular organisation. If you meet a person you do not know, you should ask for proof of identity before passing on any information.

Carers and relatives

There are over six million carers in the UK. Of course, not all of them are caring for someone with dementia, but many of them are. Generally, people who care for relatives or friends do so willingly and with love; some find it stressful and are doing it because they feel they have been forced into the situation, but this is rare. Caring is hard work and can be very stressful. Looking after someone with dementia is very demanding and can be frustrating and infuriating, especially as family carers do not get to go home at the end of the shift. Being a full-time carer can make it difficult to access some of the opportunities that are available to other people, such as education, employment and health and social care. Legislation is seeking to address the issues faced by carers.

Carers' rights in Scotland

Scotland has a Charter of Rights for people with dementia and their carers. These rights can be summarised as follows:

- participation in decisions that affect their human rights

- accountability of those responsible for the respect, protection and fulfilment of the human rights of people with dementia and their carers
- non-discrimination and equality
- empowerment to know their rights and how to claim them (for example, the right to access education, social and legal services and health and social care services)
- legality: the right to the same civil and legal rights as everyone else, particularly regarding interventions on people who lack capacity.

Refer to the Further reading and research section at the end of this chapter to find out more about the Charter of Rights.

Carers' rights in the rest of the UK

In recent years, legislation in other parts of the UK has provided some support and rights for carers. There are two aspects to carers' legal rights: those that relate to carers and those that relate to the person they are caring for.

Carers' rights include:

- the right to have their own needs assessed by the local authority
- the right to receive direct payments so that they can chose what services to have
- rights in the workplace.

Assessment of the needs of carers

Carers' rights to an assessment of their needs is set out in the Carers and Disabled Children Act 2000. This states that all carers aged 16 or above, who provide a 'regular and substantial amount of care' for someone aged 18 or over, have the right to an assessment of their needs as a carer from their local Social Services Department.

If there is more than one carer providing regular care in a household, both are entitled to an assessment.

The Carers (Equal Opportunities) Act 2005 ensures that carers have to be made aware of their right to an assessment. It also states that the carers' needs must be taken into account when undertaking an assessment. This means that if the carer has needs such as wanting to train in order to return to employment, wanting to learn to drive or any training, education, employment or leisure-related needs, these can be met as a result of the assessment.

Direct payments to carers

Direct payments are available to carers to support them to employ the services they need to assist them in their caring role. Many carers prefer to organise and employ support workers themselves, rather than have a service provided by the local authority.

Rights in the workplace

Carers who are employed have the right to ask for flexible working if they live with the person they care for. Employers are not bound to grant these requests. However, they must give business reasons for refusing a request for flexible working.

Carers also have the right to take unpaid time off work in an emergency relating to the person they care for.

The Equality Act 2010 gives carers the same protection from discrimination as the person they care for. This means that in matters such as the buying of goods and services, including shops, leisure facilities and access, the carer is also protected by the law against being treated any less favourably than someone who is not a carer.

Acting with the cared-for person's consent

The legal position in relation to the person with dementia is that as long as the person with dementia has capacity to make decisions, then they are in control of their own life and a carer can only act with the person's consent. However, if a Lasting Power of Attorney (LPA) has been put in place while the person still had capacity, then the carer can take the decisions identified in the LPA. If the person lacks capacity, and there is no LPA in place, the Court of Protection can appoint the carer as a deputy to enable them to make decisions in the person's best interests.

It is essential that all professionals work closely with family carers and that they are involved in all decisions regardless of the legal status. However, it is important to be clear that this can only be done with the consent of the person with dementia as long as they have capacity. It is not acceptable to discuss anything with a carer if the person with dementia does not agree to this.

Sharing information with carers

There is a balance to be reached with family carers of someone with dementia. They are the main part of the team providing the support to the person, so refusing to share information in those circumstances is very difficult. It is like being unable to share information with other professionals. Usually, the person concerned is willing for information to be shared with family members who are providing care and support, so this resolves the problem.

On the rare occasions when this permission is refused, you will not be able to share confidential information. Obviously, if there are problems of this nature with carers, it may be that this is not a situation in which the person is happy and they may wish to consider options for alternative living arrangements.

Relatives will often claim that they have a 'right to know'. The most famous example of this was when Victoria Gillick went to court in order to try to gain access to her daughter's medical records. She claimed that she had the right to know whether her daughter, who was under 16, had been given the contraceptive pill. Her GP had refused to tell her and she took the case all the way to the House of Lords, but the ruling was not changed and she was not given access to her daughter's records. The rules remain the same. Even for close relatives, the information is not available unless the individual agrees.

It is difficult, however, if you are faced with angry or distressed relatives who believe that you have information they are entitled to – if you encounter a son or daughter, for example, who believes that they have the right to be told about medical information regarding their parent. The best response is to be clear and assertive, but to demonstrate that you understand it is difficult for them. For example, you could say, 'I'm sorry. I know you must be worried, but I can't discuss any information unless your mother agrees.'

Activity 4

Find out about the confidentiality policies in your workplace. Check out the rules on obtaining agreement from people before sharing information, even with carers. Find out how people should be told about their rights to confidentiality.

Review the policies and see if you feel they are effective in respecting people's right to confidentiality. Write down any change you think would make the policies better.

2: Be able to maximise the rights and choices of people with dementia

2.1 Considering best interests

The Mental Capacity Act 2005 (MCA) requires that any decisions that have to be taken on behalf of an individual because they lack capacity must be 'in the person's best interests'. The person's interests take priority over those of other people, such as family, other patients or residents or the general public.

The MCA does not set out a process for making decisions, as the types of decisions are so varied. It does set out what needs to be taken into consideration in the Best Interests checklist. Anyone who is taking a decision in the best interests of someone who lacks capacity must comply with this checklist.

Best Interests checklist

- The decision must not be made merely on the basis of the person's age or appearance. In other words, a proper assessment of capacity must have been carried out.

- The person's behaviour should not lead to assumptions about what might be in their best interests. All aspects of a decision and potential consequences should be considered and reasons for any behaviour must also be considered.

- All relevant circumstances need to be considered. All aspects of someone's life and present circumstances should be taken into account.

- Is the person likely to regain capacity? Can the decision wait? Regaining capacity is unlikely in the case of someone with dementia, although the question must be asked.

- Involve the person in the decision making as much as possible. Even though it has been determined that the individual lacks capacity to make this decision, their views need to be considered and the process needs to include them as far as possible. All efforts to use various means of communication should be used to try to get the person's views as far as possible.

- If the decision concerns life-sustaining treatment, the decision must not be based on a desire to bring about death. The MCA cannot be used for the purposes of euthanasia. In other words, if a person is on life support, best interest decision making cannot be used to decide to end the life support.

- The decision maker must consider the person's past and present wishes, beliefs and values that would influence their decision making if they had capacity and any other factors the person would take into consideration if making their own decision. This is where any advance decisions made be the person can be useful, as these can help the decision maker to understand what the person is most likely to want. See below for more on advance decisions.

- The decision maker must take into account the views of anyone who cares for the person or who is interested in their welfare – this includes both paid and informal carers. The decision maker must consult, if possible, anyone who has a Lasting Power of Attorney or who is a deputy appointed by the Court of Protection. All of those who are involved with the person should be included if at all possible. Sometimes people will have useful information that was not known previously, or they may have an insight that others have missed. It is important to remember that people are being involved to get their views of what is likely to be in the best interests of the person – it is not about what is in the best interests of carers.

All of these principles are important when delivering care and support. When you act in someone's best interests, it does not mean just doing whatever you think may be best for them. You must take everything into account, including any advance decisions, or anything you know about what the person would have wanted and how they would have preferred their care and support to be delivered. The progressive nature of dementia means that you may begin to support someone at a stage when they are able to be clear about what they want, so you will be able to use this knowledge as the dementia progresses to help you to be sure that you are taking the person's wishes into account.

2.2 and 2.3 Making decisions

The principles of the Mental Capacity Act include the important concept that everyone is assumed to have the capacity to make decisions unless there is evidence that they do not. It is also important to remember that the Act states that people can only be found to lack capacity for a specific decision; lacking capacity for one particular decision does not mean that they are incapable of making any decisions. For example, someone may be very capable of deciding what to eat or what to wear, but may not be able to manage their finances.

People with dementia may need support to make decisions, but that does not mean that they should not make them. All possible support should be provided. This could include support with communication, such as using flash cards, or using an advocate to explain the person's wishes. Making decisions is part of every person's life; it gives people dignity and is part of our rights as a human being. Being in control of our own lives is good for our self-esteem and overall well-being, so being able to make decisions for as long as possible is very important.

The following comments are from people with dementia about how they feel when decisions are made for them:

'It sometimes seemed that the minute my back was turned, something else would be done without any consultation and always with the comment that it was for my own good and that I had been told what was going on.'

'When my family said "you can't go" it made me angry. I am capable of doing so much. I have forethought and foresight to know if I can't do a challenge.'

Making advance decisions

Some people may want to prepare certain decisions in advance, before the dementia progresses to the point where they are no longer able to do so. When someone makes advance decisions they should be recorded so that they can be referred to later. Such decisions may concern types of medical treatment or where a person wishes to be supported to live. They may also identify priorities for how the person wants future care and support to be provided and also how they wish their end-of-life care to be given. Advance decisions are a helpful way of involving people in decision making and of making sure that their wishes taken into account, even after they have passed the stage of being able to make decisions independently.

Case study

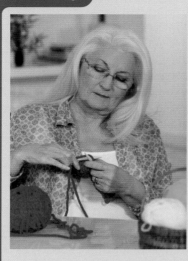

Marjorie is in the early stages of dementia. She has researched what is likely to happen and understands how the stages of dementia are likely to progress. She is currently very able to make all her own decisions and she has continues to do so. She has chosen to remain in her own home and is supported by a mix of family and friends. For the moment, she does not need the support of professional carers, but she has decided to go to the day centre for a day each week as she wants to get to know other people in a similar situation to herself. She is also happy to spend time on her own and still enjoys meeting up with friends and listening to music, watching old films and doing her own gardening. She no longer knits using patterns, as she finds the patterns confusing, but has been knitting some squares for the local church.

Marjorie has sat down with her children and prepared some advance decisions about what she wants to happen later. She has decided that she will only go into residential care at the point where she is at risk living at home and she is happy that her son and daughter will be able to make this decision if she is unable to. Her preference would be to remain at home with professional support. At this point, she does not think that she would want to be resuscitated if she were to develop a life-threatening condition.

1 Do you think it is helpful for Marjorie to write down her decisions in advance?

2 Who will benefit from her doing this?

3 How do you think Marjorie feels about being able to make advance decisions?

One of the principles of behaving in someone's best interests is that, whatever action needs to be taken, it must give people as much freedom as possible and must limit their lives as little as possible. Examples of this are given in the following case studies about Tom and June.

Case study

Tom likes to go out walking every day, but he often gets lost. The last time he went out he was picked up by the police, as he was walking down the approach road to the motorway. Tom is moving towards an advanced stage of dementia, but becomes very distressed if he does not get to walk each day.

A decision needs to be taken in Tom's best interests about if, or how, he is to be able to go out for walks.

In this case, the least restrictive option would be for Tom to have his daily walk with an assistant to support him and ensure that he returns safely. Tom could be made to stay in, but that would be very restrictive and definitely a decision he would oppose if he were able.

1 Do you think these were the least restrictive options?

2 What else could have been considered?

3 Why is it important to look for the least restrictive option?

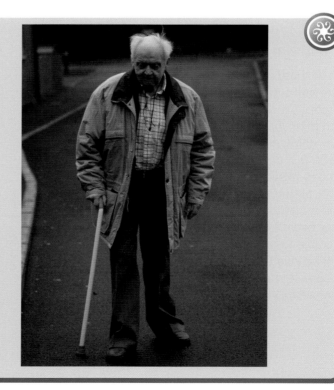

Case study

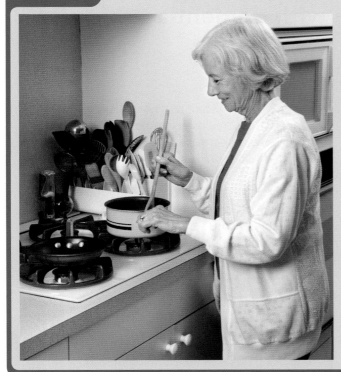

June lives at home and has support from family and professional carers. She has always been adamant that she wished to remain in her own home, and she made this clear in her advance decisions and care priorities when she was able. Her dementia is progressing. On several occasions recently, she has left the gas cooker turned on but unlit. Neighbours are supportive but they are concerned, as she lives in a terraced house. The options being discussed are:

- a move to a residential home
- a move to extra care housing
- replacing her gas cooker with an electric one
- turning off the gas to the cooker and providing prepared meals for the microwave.

The social worker and her family decided on the last option. This was felt to be the least restrictive way to support June.

1   Do you think these were the least restrictive options?

2   What else could have been considered?

3   Why is it important to look for the least restrictive option?

Activity 5

Choose someone you support who does not have the capacity to make their own decisions in some areas of their life. Think about a decision that has been made on their behalf. Look at the different options for the solutions to the concerns ane make notes about what they were. Note the following questions and find the answer to each of them.

1   Were all options considered?

2   Was the least restrictive option chosen?

3   What were the alternatives?

4   Would they have all been more restrictive for the person?

5   Why?

2.4 Fluctuating ability to make decisions

One of the difficulties for people with dementia is that their condition can be changeable. Dementia is not a constant condition, and how people are on a particular day can be the result of a range of factors. Sometimes the factors can be physical, such as:

- not feeling well
- being in pain
- being tired
- effects of medication
- being hot or cold
- being uncomfortable
- constipation.

Emotions can also affect how well people can understand and retain the information necessary for the decision-making process, such as:

- feeling anxious
- feeling depressed
- being frustrated
- being angry.

Each of these factors, or a combination of them, can mean that a person who was able to discuss the aspects of a decision one day may not even remember the question the following day, or a week later. Recording information about people's wishes and decisions is important, so that you know what they want and can use the information to act in their best interests if necessary.

3: Involving carers of people with dementia

3.1 Involving carers in planning

When developing a support plan for a person with dementia, a self-assessment will have been carried out by the person and their carer to reach an agreement about what support can be provided by friends, family and the community and what services are needed to fill the gaps. You may be involved at the stage of making the plan, or you may only become involved at the stage of putting the support plan into action. Regardless of when your role begins, you need to be clear about the assessment process, which is as follows.

- The person and their carer should be full partners in both assessment and planning.
- Carers are often the best people to give information about the person's strengths and abilities and to identify what they are able to do for themselves.
- The full range of needs that the person identifies must be taken into account.
- Information must be available in a variety of formats, so that the person and their carer are able to take a full part in the process.
- Separate assessments must be offered to carers of their own needs.
- People who lack the capacity to participate in the assessment and planning process should have their carer and/or advocate as fully involved as possible to act in their best interests.

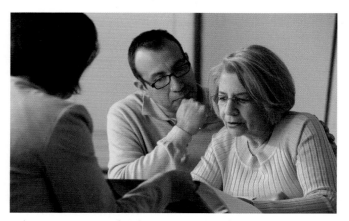

Why is it important for the carer to be a full partner in assessment and planning as well as the person they are supporting?

Meetings with social care professionals can be very intimidating for some carers and they may not have the confidence to participate. It is important that you encourage the person, their carer and their family, and any friends they wish to be involved, to feel able to make an active and effective contribution to the planning process. Planning meetings are all about the person with dementia, and their carers are often the most important people to them. It is possible to lose sight of this and to allow the carer to feel that their role is purely a passive one.

Doing it well

Supporting carers in the planning process

There are several actions that you can take to support the carer to recognise that they have a useful and important contribution to make to the planning process.

1. Go through the procedure of the planning process with them so that they know what will happen, in what order information will be discussed and the type of contributions that they may be asked to make.
2. Give carers the opportunity to prepare in advance what they want to say and to work out the best way to present it. They might prefer to present their contribution in a written form or they could prepare some notes in advance to ensure that they cover all the points they want to make.
3. Make sure they know the options available for a support plan and how the Resource Allocation System will be used to work out how much money will be available for their budget. In this way, they will not be surprised by any of the decisions that could be made. Explain to them that there could be a range of options to consider.
4. Where necessary, make practical arrangements for them to participate. This could include ensuring accessibility, providing transport or providing translation or other communication assistance.

Try to remember situations in which you felt you were not in control and that other people held the power. Examples could include:

- an appointment with a doctor in which you felt unable to ask all the questions that you wanted to because the doctor did not seem to have time to answer them
- a situation that involved lawyers or other professionals
- a meeting with your child's teacher or head teacher who made you feel you were lacking in the skill and ability to put across what you really wanted to say.

Remember how you felt in those situations and think about how much easier it might have been if somebody had been supporting you. Choose one of the situations to act as your 'trigger' to recall those feelings whenever you are in a support planning meeting, or any other situation, with a person with dementia and/or their carer. This should remind you to encourage people to put across their views if they are having difficulty doing so.

Checking support planning decisions

Any proposals for a support plan must reflect the wishes of the person with dementia, and their family carer should also be happy with the proposed plan. It is important that you seek out the carer's confirmation of the agreement even if the carer was present at the planning meeting. This is important for two reasons:

1 They will have had time to reflect and think things over since the planning meeting and their views may have changed.

2 They might not have felt able to express any reservations that they may have had during the meeting.

You will need to make sure you give carers the opportunity to express any doubts or concerns they have at this stage. It is always more helpful to establish concerns before a plan has begun than to have to adapt and change the service during its provision. It is important that those who are involved with the care of a person with dementia are given the opportunity to comment on the proposals and the extent to which they believe that the service will meet the person's needs and their own needs.

You will need to explain the process clearly so that carers understand how the process works and their role in it. You will also need to work actively to check out any possible barriers and make sure that they are overcome. The kind of barriers which can prevent carers becoming involved in effectively planning and monitoring support are:

- using jargon and complex professional language
- making the process complicated and difficult to understand
- having an attitude which might intimidate or alienate carers
- designing a planning system using methods which are not the preferred means of communication for the person concerned.

Carers should be involved at every stage of the planning, monitoring, review and evaluation of services, and you should use a checklist at the different stages of the process to ensure that you have covered all the potential barriers and found ways to overcome them.

3.2 Conflicts between carers and the person with dementia

There may be disagreements between a person with dementia and members of their family or close friends about the type or amount of support or the way in which support should be provided. It may be useful to provide all those who are involved with a copy of the support plan, with space for them to make notes about whether they agree or disagree with the proposals and to make any comments that they have. Sometimes being able to write things down can help people to reflect and consider the issues they have.

Ultimately, your responsibility is to the person with dementia. It is to them that you have a duty of care. However, you also have a responsibility towards the person's carers and to try to resolve differences of opinion, although this can sometimes be difficult. Most disagreements result from families being protective and wanting to ensure that their loved one is not exposed to risk, whereas the person with dementia may want to be involved in activities or to make arrangements that give them more independence, thus exposing themselves to greater risks. In these situations, remember the underlying principles of working with people with dementia: it is their right to make their own choices and decisions and to take risks if they want to as long as they have the capacity to make the decision.

Sometimes, carers can feel that someone does not have capacity to make decisions, but a capacity assessment may come up with a different outcome. It is not always easy for loving families to accept that just because a decision seems foolish or unreasonable, this is not sufficient reason to decide that a person does not have the capacity to make it. It can be a delicate task to explain this to carers.

Of course, there may be situations where the conflict with carers is not based on loving concern, but on their own personal gain. For example, a family may consistently try to keep a person with dementia in their own home rather than in residential care because they do not wish to have the cost of residential care taken from the value of a property that they will inherit. In these circumstances, you will need to take any necessary steps to act in the best interests of the person with dementia.

3.3 Supporting people to complain

Complaints to an organisation are an important part of the monitoring process and they should be considered as part of every review of service provision. If everyone simply puts up with poor service and no one complains, the service providers will never become aware of where the service needs improvement. Similarly, if complaints are not responded to appropriately, services will never improve. All service providers or organisations that commission services will have a system for complaints.

There will be clear information about how and to whom a complaint should be made and timescales for it to be dealt with.

An important part of exercising rights is being able to complain if services are poor or do not meet expectations. All public service organisations are required to have a complaints procedure and to make the procedure readily available for people to use. Part of your role may be to assist service users in making complaints, either directly by supporting them in following the procedure, or indirectly by making sure that they are aware of the complaints procedure and are able to follow it. Most complaints procedures will involve an informal stage, where complaints are discussed before they become more formal issues.

People with dementia and their carers can find themselves the subject of decisions made by professionals. They may not agree with the decisions, but may not always feel able to challenge them. Decisions could be about:

- accommodation
- the support plan
- changes in service provision
- an assessment
- medication
- development activities
- personal care
- leisure time.

Case study

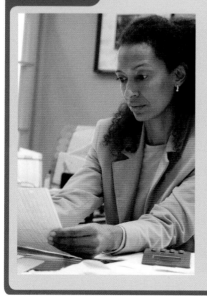

Julie is an assistant director in a local authority with responsibility for commissioning services for older people. She has recently been receiving a series of complaints about a particular day care facility. The complaints are different: one or two have been about transport being late, a couple about the quality of the food and most recently one about the attitudes of staff. This has made Julie decide to ask the service manager to carry out a review of the facility and to look at what is going wrong. Seen separately, these isolated complaints may have gone unnoticed, but when put together they suggest a picture of a provision that is not working as it should.

1   What could have happened if Julie had not asked for a review of the service?
2   Why is it important to learn lessons from complaints?
3   What were the advantages of seeing a wider picture?
4   How could these issues have been dealt with separately?
5   How could you make sure that information from complaints is not lost?

Although good practice requires that people with dementia should always be in control of decisions, this does not always happen. Sometimes events just happen, such as the closure of a facility, new decisions about financial spending or changes in family circumstances. Sometimes it is the nature of the decision that does not put the person or their carer in control, for example, decisions about benefits, immigration status or employment issues. In some cases, it may just be as a result of poor practice!

People can find it hard to challenge a decision that has been made for them. It can be difficult for a range of reasons, including:

- people feel intimidated
- people lack the confidence to make a challenge
- people do not believe that they have the right to challenge the decisions of professionals
- people may have had poor experiences in the past when they have challenged decisions unsuccessfully
- people may simply not know how to go about it.

People with dementia and/or their carers can be supported to overcome all of these barriers. You may be able to provide encouragement and also practical help and advice. The case study below about Hassan illustrates how someone can be supported in exercising their rights to question and challenge decisions.

Everyone should be able to complain about poor service, regardless of what the service is and who is providing it. People with dementia and their carers should be encouraged to recognise that any organisation which operates to high standards will welcome complaints and use them as part of their process for monitoring and improving their services. You should make it clear to people that if they have any problems with any services as a result of complaining, this would raise concerns about the quality of the service and would need to be investigated.

Case study

Hassan's doctor decided to change his medication. Hassan was unhappy about it as he felt this was unnecessary, but did not feel that he could argue with the doctor. Hassan has been diagnosed with dementia, but he is the early stages and he is coping well. Carole, his support worker, spent time with Hassan to talk through his worries and encouraged him to write some notes explaining his concerns. She then agreed to go with Hassan to see the doctor, but only to support him while he raised the issues himself. In the event, Carole did not need to say a word. Hassan used his notes to explain to his doctor why he was unhappy and disagreed with the change. Even when the doctor got quite impatient, Hassan was still able to stay focused and make his point.

1 Was this a good solution?
2 What were the key reasons why Hassan was able to do this?
3 What might have happened if Hassan had not spoken to the doctor?

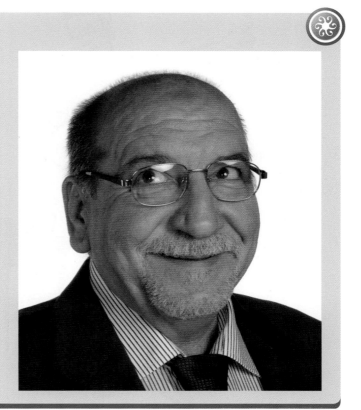

4: How to maintain privacy, dignity and respect and promote choice

Everyone is entitled to be treated with dignity and respect in all aspects of life, from support with personal care to how people want to be addressed. Treating people with dignity and respect also involves listening to what people have to say and being interested in them. Sometimes people with dementia do not get the respect they deserve, nor do they get treated with dignity because it is all too easy to assume that 'they won't know any different'.

Not only is this far from the truth, but even if it were accurate for some people, being unaware of your surroundings does not make poor and unprofessional attitudes acceptable. In fact, people who struggle to grasp the world around them deserve even more care and consideration.

4.1 Privacy for personal care

Everyone has a right to have some space where they can be alone if they wish. Sometimes they may want to be private just to have some time to themselves; on other occasions they may need privacy they are receiving personal care or medical treatment. It is also important that people have privacy if they want to talk to a professional and have confidential information to discuss.

Ideally people should be able to manage their personal care independently and in private. However, this is not always possible as some people with dementia may need some degree of assistance. How much someone can manage unaided is likely to change over time as the

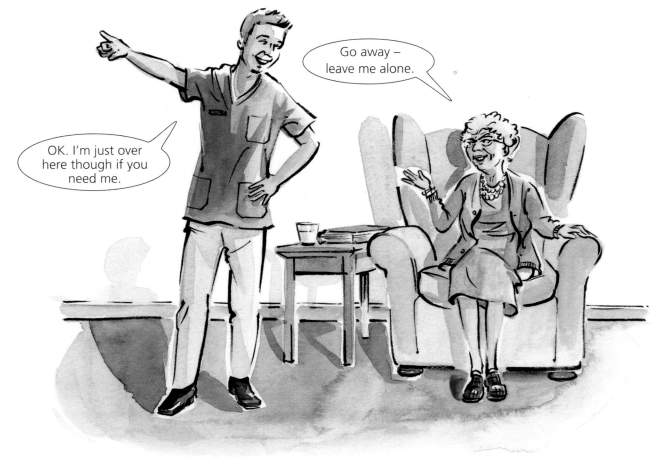

Figure 5.4: How is this carer demonstrating good practice?

dementia progresses. The level of assistance required will need to be kept under constant review in consultation with the person and any family or friend carers.

Sometimes it can be risky for the person to manage personal care for themselves unsupervised – for example, someone may struggle to remain focused on what they are doing and forget to get fully dressed or they may forget to check the temperature of a bath or shower. People may be unable to recall the right order for putting on clothes or may forget to clean themselves properly after using the toilet. In the early stages of dementia, this is less likely to be a problem, but as time passes it is important to change the levels of support.

Doing it well

If support is needed and agreed, then you must work in a sensitive way. Try to empathise with the person's situation. Simple actions can maximise privacy and make all the difference, for example, knocking on the door before entering the room.

Maintaining a person's privacy can be more difficult in a hospital setting where there may only be a curtain around the bed, but you can make sure that there are no gaps in the curtains and alert the person by calling their name and asking permission to enter before opening the curtains.

If someone is being supported with personal care at home and they are unable to use their bathroom (for example, it may be upstairs and they have limited mobility), then you can ensure that privacy is maintained by closing curtains or blinds and making sure that the room door is closed to prevent people outside from seeing the activity.

Modesty is greatly valued by some religions and cultural groups. Talk to the person and their family in order to check the level of privacy required by someone's religion or culture when personal care is being undertaken.

If someone requires full support for personal care, maximum privacy can still be maintained. For example, if the person needs help with an assisted wash or a blanket bath, use extra towels or a warm sheet to ensure that they remain covered as much as possible.

Reflect

Imagine that you are a patient in a hospital and you share a bay with five other people. There are people of the opposite sex on the ward in other bays. You have had an operation and are unable to manage your own personal care, so you need someone to help you.

How you would feel in this situation? How would you like to be supported?

4.2 Physical aspects of the environment

Where people live has just as much impact on well-being as how people live. When someone has dementia, living in the right environment, which has a well thought-out design, can make a significant difference to how well they can function. Considerable work has been undertaken by architects and designers to look at how to get the best environment for people with dementia. There are some basic, internationally agreed principles that the design of care facilities should:

- compensate for impairments
- maximise independence
- enhance self-esteem and confidence
- be understandable and not confusing
- reinforce people's identity
- not be over-stimulating.

Compensate for impairments

The thinking behind this principle is that an impairment only becomes a disability if the design of a living space does not overcome the impairment. For example, as people with dementia may have impaired memory, creating an open-plan design so that all areas can be seen and so eating areas and sitting areas are easily located can assist people to feel comfortable and familiar with their surroundings. Toilet doors should always be in the same colour that is a good contrast to the surrounding walls. Signs should be large and clear. In en-suite bathrooms, the toilet should be clearly visible from the bed. These things may sound like small details but they all assist people to live well with dementia.

People with dementia are also likely to have impaired reasoning and find it difficult to make judgements and to process information. People can lose the ability to tell the difference between colours, so sharp contrasts are important. Difficulties in recognising colours usually starts with blue, purple and green. Red, orange and yellow are recognised for the longest, so these can be good colours to choose. Design features that can help include:

- clear contrasts between surfaces and objects
- clear contrast between floor and wall finishes and between handrails and grab rails and the walls behind
- light switches that contrast clearly with the background,
- a toilet seat that contrasts with the toilet, which in turn contrasts with the background floor and wall tiling.

A sharp contrast in flooring colour can be perceived as a step by people with dementia, so similar colours in flooring should be used, but different textures between hard floor and carpet can indicate the different areas.

When people have impaired orientation, it has been found that architectural features, rather than colour, can often be the most helpful way for people to find their way around. Curved walls, different textures for wall coverings or features such as clocks or plants should be individual so that people find it easier to know where they are.

Maximise independence

A well-designed environment can help people to make the most of their independence by giving them the opportunity to safely explore and move around the building. Many people with dementia like to walk, and providing indoor or outdoor areas for safe walking can help people to be independent and make their own choices about when and where they will walk. Areas such as exit doors can be painted to match surrounding walls and removing features such as door frames can reduce the risks of people wandering out of the premises.

Enhance self-esteem

People's self-esteem can be improved by supporting them to maintain their skills. Kitchen work surfaces that can be adjusted to different heights and careful thought given to the kitchen layout can help with this. The option for residents to contribute to the running of their own household by undertaking everyday tasks is important in maintaining a continuation of their everyday life. In some

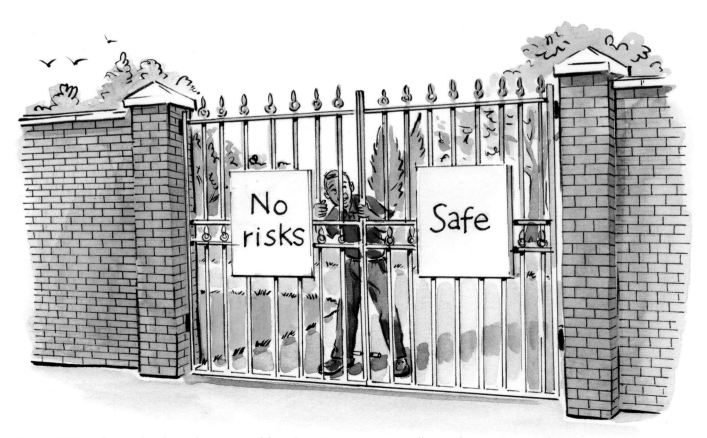

Figure 5.5: Independence and a sense of freedom is important to all people

residential facilities, the kitchenettes in the care home households are accessible to residents, and the residents and staff make meals, snacks and drinks together. Dementia should not prevent people from being active in their community. Residential or extra care facilities should be able to use garden areas and community rooms for clubs and groups to meet.

Recognise individual identity

Rooms that help to maintain people's identity are important. People should be able to have their own belongings around them and the opportunity to have memory boxes around the door area helps people to recognise their own room and also gives others information about who lives there.

Levels of stimulation

It is important that there is a calm and relaxed atmosphere in a living environment for people with dementia. Too many different 'busy' and noisy features can add to confusion and anxiety. It is easy for people with dementia to be over-stimulated by too many bright colours, bright and harsh lighting and too much noise. Using floor coverings that are quiet to walk on and providing quiet and peaceful areas are ways of achieving a calm and relaxing environment for people.

Activity 6

Look at the design principles listed above. Now apply each one of them to your workplace. How well does your workplace match up? Is there more that could be done? What could be improved and how would you go about doing this? Make notes and draw some plans of what you would like to do. You could research and put together photographs of rooms and designs that you think would improve the living environment of the people you support.

If you work with people in their own homes, design a new residential or extra care facility.

4.3 Social aspects of the environment

Supporting people with dementia means providing a social environment that encourages people to do as much as they can for themselves and to make their own choices about how they wish to live, not imposing routines on them.

The overall atmosphere should be calm and relaxed and provide people with a feeling of warmth, security and caring. This type of environment will help people with dementia to feel less anxious and confused and more orientated and focused and, therefore, better able to participate and maintain skills and intellectual functioning.

Providing a caring and secure environment is very important, but that does not mean that people should have everything done for them. Giving people the opportunity to make choices and take risks is an important part of supporting people to reach their potential. Everyone should be encouraged to do as much as they possibly can for themselves. It is likely that the more they are encouraged, the more they will be able to achieve.

Participating in activities with others and achieving goals usually helps people to feel good about themselves and improves confidence and self-esteem. How we value ourselves is key to our sense of well-being. Helping people to feel good and confident are important ways of improving people's general and emotional health. This is no less true for people with dementia: feeling self-confident and independent is just as important.

It is tempting to do things *for* people because this may be easier, quicker and less difficult and it may seem that this is be the most helpful thing to do. In fact, doing tasks for people is far from helpful as it results in people becoming de-skilled and increases dependency. Increasing people's dependency will decrease their confidence, self-esteem and sense of well-being, leading to people becoming depressed and feeling isolated.

Encourage people to undertake as much of their personal care as they can possible manage, including hygiene, managing their own appearance, choosing clothes and keeping themselves clean. Obviously, the level of ability to do this will vary with the stage of dementia and will change over time, but people should always do the absolute maximum that they can.

Working *with* people to support them where there are things that they really cannot do for themselves is so much better than taking over and doing tasks for people and making them dependent on you.

Reflect

Think about someone you support. Identify a task or activity that is carried out for them. Why are they unable to do this task themselves? Is there anything more that could be done to support them to do this for themselves?

Getting ready for assessment

This unit is all about balancing rights and risks, so you will have to show that you understand why it is necessary for people to be able to take risks in order to exercise their rights to make choices about their lives. Your assessor will want to see that you have understood how legislation and policies create the framework for supporting people with dementia to make choices and exercise rights.

DEM 304 is a competence unit that requires knowledge and demonstration of skills. You will need to demonstrate in a workplace setting that you are able to involve people and their carers and families in their own support. This means that you must be able to show that people have chosen their support package as far as possible, and that families and friends have been involved to assist with this. You will need to be able to show your assessor that you are able to work in the best interests of a person with dementia when they lack capacity to make decisions, and that you support people who can make decisions to do so. Your assessor will want to know what you do in your practice to make sure that people's rights are respected and they are able to make choices and decisions about their lives.

When you are asked to explain, do not simply list or describe. Use words such as 'because', 'as a result of', 'so that' and 'in order to'. If you are explaining something you must show that you understand the reasons for it. Where you are asked to evaluate, you will need to weigh the options and alternatives, and reach a conclusion that is clearly supported by evidence.

Further reading and research

- www.cqc.org.uk (Care Quality Commission: responsible for inspecting social care facilities in England).
- www.dementiarights.org (charter of rights for people with dementia and their carers in Scotland).
- www.equalityhumanrights.com (Equality and Human Rights Commission: this works to challenge discrimination and to protect and promote human rights. Use the website's search facility to find out about how the work of the Commission applies to people with dementia).
- www.rqia.org.uk (Regulation and Quality Improvement Authority: responsible for inspecting social care facilities in Northern Ireland).
- www.scswis.com (Care Inspectorate: responsible for inspecting social care facilities in Scotland).
- www.un.org (United Nations: click on the 'Human Rights' tab and then follow the link to the Universal Declaration of Human Rights to see the full text of the Declaration).
- www.wales.gov.uk/cssiwsubsite/newcssiw/?lang=en (Care and Social Services Inspectorate Wales: responsible for inspecting social care facilities in Wales).

Glossary

Advocacy – speaking on someone's behalf to help them get what they need.

Civil – relating to ordinary citizens and their concerns.

Delirium – severe confusion, involving rapid changes between different mental states and disorganised thinking.

Delusions – believing things that are not real.

Discrimination – treating a group of people differently from others, usually treating them in a worse way.

Diversity – the differences between people.

Duty of care – a legal obligation to do everything you can to keep those in your care safe from harm.

Empathy – the ability to understand and share the feelings of someone else.

Goodwill – the established reputation of a business regarded as an asset.

Hallucinations – seeing things that are not really there.

Oppression – using a position of power to keep people down or to treat them badly.

PEG (Percutaneous Endoscopic Gastronomy) feeding – a means of giving people nutrition directly into the stomach. It is used when people are unable to swallow.

Protected characteristic – these include age, disability, gender reassignment, marriage and civil partnership, pregnancy and maternity, race, religion and belief, sex and sexual orientation.

Psychosis – an episode when someone is out of touch with reality.

Public body – an organisation whose work is part of the process is government, but which is not a government department.

Self-esteem – how you value yourself, and therefore how you believe the rest of the world sees you.

Self-image/self-concept – how people see themselves.

Statutory – required, permitted or created by law.

Tribunal – a special court convened by government to inquire into a specific matter.

Further reading and research

Websites

Action for Advocacy
www.actionforadvocacy.org.uk
Information on all types of advocacy, what each does and how to access an advocate.

Alzheimer's Research UK
www.alzheimersresearchUK.org
The UK's leading dementia research charity.

Alzheimer's Society
www.alzheimers.org.uk
The UK's leading care and research charity for individuals with dementia and those who care for them. The organisation provides information, support, guidance and referrals to other appropriate organisations. The website also has plenty of information on communicating with people who have dementia.

AT Dementia
www.atdementia.org.uk
An organisation that provides information on assistive technology that can help people with dementia live more independently. It is particularly useful for information about using equipment to aid medication.

British Institute of Learning Disabilities
www.bild.org.uk
Works to improve the lives of individuals with disabilities. It provides a range of published and online information.

British National Formulary
www.bnf.org
Contains information about all medicines.

Care and Social Services Inspectorate Wales
www.wales.gov.uk/cssiwsubsite/newcssiw/?lang=en
This organisation is responsible for inspecting social care facilities in Wales.

Care Inspectorate
www.scswis.com
This organisation is responsible for inspecting social care facilities in Scotland.

Care Quality Commission
www.cqc.org.uk
This organisation is responsible for inspecting social care facilities in England.

Careers Trust
www.carers.org
A new charity formed following the merger of The Princess Royal Trust for Carers and Crossroads Care. The website includes resources that focus on family carers for people who have dementia.

CJD Support
www.cjdsupport.net
An organisation which supports individuals with prion diseases, including forms of Creutzfeldt-Jakob disease (CJD). They provide a range of information on the

various forms of prion disease, and work with professionals to improve the level of care provided for individuals with these conditions.

Dementia Action Alliance

www.dementiaaction.org.uk
An organisation that brings together many organisations committed to working with dementia.

Dementia Positive

www.dementiapositive.co.uk
Useful resources on how to approach dementia in a positive and constructive way, as a result of the work of John Killick and Kate Allan.

Dementia Research Centre

www.dementia.ion.ucl.ac.uk
One of the UK's leading centres for clinical research into dementia and for trialling new drugs to slow the progression of Alzheimer's disease.

Dementia Rights

www.dementiarights.org
Charter of rights for people with dementia and their carers in Scotland.

Department of Health

Has a number of useful documents, including:

- www.dh.gov.uk/en/Healthcare/Medicinespharmacyandindustry/Prescriptions/ TheNon-MedicalPrescribingProgramme – information on prescribers who are not doctors, dentists or vets. These can include pharmacists, midwives and nurses

- www.dh.gov.uk/en/Publichealth/Scientificdevelopmentgeneticsandbioethics/ Consent/Consentgeneralinformation/index.htm – further information about consent and key documents relating to consent to treatment forms and guidance.

- www.dh.gov.uk/en/Publicationsandstatistics/Publications/ PublicationsPolicyAndGuidance/DH_094058 – Living well with dementia: A National Dementia Strategy.

Equality and Human Rights Commission

www.equalityhumanrights.com
This organisation works to challenge discrimination and to protect and promote human rights. Use the website's search facility to find out about how the work of the Commission applies to people with dementia.

General Medical Council

www.gmc-uk.org
Information on the responsibilities of doctors in relation to prescribing medicines.

Huntington's Disease Association

www.hda.org.uk
An association that provides information, advice, support and useful publications for families affected by Huntington's disease in England and Wales. It can put you in touch with a regional advisor and your nearest branch or support group.

Medicine and Healthcare products Regulatory Agency

www.mhra.gov.uk/Safetyinformation/Healthcareproviders/Carehomestaff/index.htm
A one-stop resource for care home staff.

MIMS
www.mims.co.uk
A drugs database that contains current information about medicines.

National Council for Palliative Care
www.ncpc.org.uk
Information about providing high-quality end-of-life care.

National Institute for Clinical Excellence (NICE)
www.nice.org.uk
Publishes guidelines on prescribing medication for people with dementia and has useful documents including:

- http://guidance.nice.org.uk/CG42 *Dementia* – A NICE–SCIE Guideline on supporting people with dementia and their carers in health and social care – National Clinical Practice Guideline Number 42

National Prescribing Centre
www.npc.nhs.uk
Provides information about the legislation relating to medicines.

Regulation and Quality Improvement Authority
www.rqia.org.uk
Responsible for inspecting social care facilities in Northern Ireland.

Royal College of Pharmacists
www.rpharms.com/support-pdfs/handlingmedsocialcare.pdf
This publication contains further information about administering and handling medication in social care settings in the 'medicines toolkit'.

Social Care Institute for Excellence
www.scie.org.uk
In their Dementia Gateway section, there are a large number of resources that support working with people who have dementia, including case studies.

United Nations
www.un.org
To read the Universal Declaration of Human Rights click on the 'Human Rights' tab and follow the link.

Books

Brooker, D. (2006) *Person-centred Dementia Care: Making Services Better*, Bradford Dementia Group Good Practice Guides, Jessica Kingsley Publishers, London and Philadelphia.

Table of unit numbers by awarding organisation

Chapter no. in this book	Unit no. in this book	Unit title	Unit accreditation no.	Edexcel unit no.	NCFE unit no.	CACHE/ OCR unit no.	C&G unit no.
1	DEM 301	Understand the process and experience of dementia	J/601/3538	13	10	DEM 301	4222–365
2	DEM 305	Understand the administration of medication to individuals with dementia using a person-centred approach	K/601/9199	14	14	DEM 305	4222–368
3	DEM 308	Understand the role of communication and interactions with individuals who have dementia	L/601/3539	15	15	DEM 308	4222–369
3	DEM 312	Understand and enable interaction and communication with individuals who have dementia	Y/601/4693	51	51	DEM 312	4222–371
4	DEM 310	Understand the diversity of individuals with dementia and the importance of inclusion	Y/601/3544	16	16	DEM 310	4222–370
4	DEM 313	Equality, diversity and inclusion in dementia care practice	F/601/4686	52	52	DEM 313	4222–372
5	DEM 304	Enable rights and choices of individuals with dementia whilst minimising risks	A/601/9191	50	50	DEM 304	4222–367

Knowledge units

Competence units

Index

Key terms are indicated by **bold** headings and page numbers.